Table of Contents

Preference

There is a substantial relationship between nutrition, functional foods and healthy ageing; the term functional foods were first used in Japan as early as 1980. All foods are functional although some food components provide more health benefits other than basic nutrition.

Examples of functional food and bio functional foods may be fortified, enriched with dietary supplements, or synthetically enhanced or grown via modified bacteria and/or fungi; Functional foods provide essential nutrients in quality necessary for maintenance, growth and development an enhance healthy physiological effects. Dietary supplements are also in the category of functional foods though food supplements constitute a different delivery system for bioactive components.

Nutriepigenomics explains how functional foods influence epigenetic modifications both histone modifications and Non-coding RNAs of the human genome while regulating health and disease. Epigenetics is dynamic the study of heritable meiotic and miotic changes in gene expression and repression functionalities that are not resultant of changes in DNA sequence; the structural epigenetic modifications that effect chromosomal histone-complex or nucleosomal tail methylation and acetylation are involved in tissue specific patterns that register and signal heritable gene expression without sequential DNA modifications.

The objectives are to introduce to the reader Nutrition, functional foods and Epigenetics with explanations of associated quantum theory and biological concepts throughout the text. There is a hypothesis within: Quantum field biological interactions and Pseudocertainty on epigenetics. Also, a system of referencing has been adopted: Glossary, Appendixes and Index for explanatory rational, the reader shall find the glossary an intriguing learning system which is referenced throughout the text. This publication is suitable for the general population with a thirst for knowledge, and for individuals with a studious interest in nutrition, functional foods, and epigenetics as methods towards healthy ageing. The reader's health is not guaranteed though functional foods combined with personalized nutrition will help towards healthy ageing.

Introduction

Epigenetics is the study of heritable and dynamic meiotic and miotic changes in gene expression and repression functionalities that are not resultant of changes in DNA sequence, the structural chromosomal modifications that effect histone complex methylation and acetylation are dynamic, involved in tissue specific patterns that register and signal heritable gene expression without sequential DNA modifications. Thus, epigenetic interactions are not always heritable as dynamic interactions of epigenetic clock reversal and biomarkers correction overtime is achievable via functional foods, food supplements and even future gene editing.

Nutritional micronutrients and functional foods have an effect via epigenetic histone modifications which do not directly affect DNA structure. Epigenetic control of gene expression constitutes three biological systems: Histone modifications, DNA methylation, and non-coding RNA repression. whereby effectors, effect the octamer histone protein amino tails that help to form a supportive nucleosol hairpin structure for the coiled DNA as shown in following text. Some external and internal environmental factors on epigenetics switch gene expression off via Methyl-groups, or on via acetyl-groups, with later discourse and further detail.

Maternal and nutritional epigenetic programming is inheritable, both intergenerational and transgenerational epigenetic inheritance, although when **gene biomarkers are in a <u>poised state</u>** genes are not expressed known as gene silencing. Therefore, functional foods combined with healthy lifestyle choices limits undesirable gene expression, further explained as follows.

Quote: - **"evolution is perpetuated via the most appropriate mutation, given internal and external environmental factors"** via chemical affinity and affinity via quantum interactions. King. J.L (2021*)*.

Epigenetics are reactive to functional foods and the above evolutionary factors, both external to the environment and internal to biological systems via hormonal signaling affinities; the evolutionary modification of histone methylation has evolved as a reactive defense mechanism against co-evolving pathogens, and for evolutionary selection of appropriate modifications.

The natural environmental complexities have co-evolved with all species throughout evolution, humans have been producing pollutants and creating environmental factors on a tremendous scale that impact all species. The environmental pollutants are vast, and issues are geo-political that far exceed this textbook, as environmental science considerations are geo-global-issues and geo-social-issues that will not be researched in detail within this particular publication.

Epigenetic nutritional micronutrients are considered - vitamins, minerals, herbs, fresh and functional foods. A knowledge of biological terms and Nutrition is assumed although, there is no recommendations for readers that have illnesses, or inheritable genomic modifications or knowledge of appropriate nutrition; referral to a specialist Nutritionist, G.P. and or a specialist Genomic-program practitioner or functional food practitioner is advised for advice and/or therapy.

Genomic-program-practitioners test and monitor epigenetic health utilising biological methods to discover personalized nutrition; initially utilizing swab and/or blood test for DNA sequencing, Genotyping, Epigenetics and other test to discover appropriate personalized nutrition. Future Genomic-program practitioners offer services for: DNA sequencing, Genotyping services, DNA synthesized products utilizing genome *(and future plasmid genetics for bacteria derived functional foods)* compilers to synthesis DNA, RNA or proteins; and bioinformatics services for pharmaceutical companies, diagnostics, also for the food and agricultural biotechnological research markets.

Chapter 1

Internal and external environmental factors on Epigenetics

Pollutants such as Bisphenol, Phthalates, Pesticides and metals... are environmental factors that have impact on both histone epigenetic alterations and genome DNA mutations; most environmental pollutants are detrimental to optimal health although debatably accepted and tolerated if the pollutants are within 'recommended levels', histone epigenetic modifications are often modified due to pollutants although antioxidants assist to diminish the detrimental free radicals. Plastics, adhesives, solvents and personal care products are all phthalates, and metals (cadmium, chromium, lead, nickel and zinc...) all have many dangerous and decremental transgenerational effects that are mostly not reversible, though synthetic biology may assist in the future with gene editing and other sustainable environmental solutions.

Gamma particles from the sun are normally filtered by stratospheric ozone (between 15-25km high), though chlorofluorocarbons (CFCs) have caused ozone-depletion ($O_3 \rightarrow O_2$) and the consequential gamma particles are often involved in epigenomic hypermethylation modifications of the skin; though vitamin D is synthesized with sunlight, discouragement with respect to sunbathing is advisable in avoidance of undesirable modifications. Other pollutants and toxins have effects on epigenetic activation and repression of gene expression and immunity, examples would be oxidative damage that occurs during metabolism because oxygen is a radical with two unpaired electrons that spin in the same direction during metabolism. Homeostasis of the oxidants, antioxidants and redox status should complete otherwise consequential imbalance occurs. This physiological unbalance is addressed through intake of nutritional antioxidants, i.e., Vitamin A, C and selenium dependent glutathione and other antioxidant enhancing functional foods.

Functional foods

The National Academy of Sciences' Food and Nutrition Board cites those functional foods is "any modified food or food ingredient that may provide a health benefit beyond the traditional nutrients it contains" (Earl R, Thomas PR (eds) (1994). and the International Life Sciences Institute cites "foods that, by virtue of the presence of physiologically-active components, provide a health benefit beyond basic nutrition". The American Dietetic Association definition of functional foods cites the same as above and acknowledges foods that are "whole, fortified, enriched, or enhanced," and consumed "as part of a varied diet on a regular basis, at effective levels" for imparting health benefits to consumers (Thomson C et al - 1999) Thus functional foods are enhanced and fortified which provide health benefits with regular nutritional value towards optimal health when taken in regular specified quantity, functional foods are considered similar to genetically modified products wherein are fortified with additional nutritional benefit of preventive measure against several diseases in order to treat the medical conditions (Weststrate JA et al -2002).

Functional foods are an important source in the prevention, management, and treatment of diseases, functional foods can be natural, processed or engineered bio functional foods that contain known bioactive micronutrients; defined as foods that have additional functions via insertion of new ingredients or enhancement of existing ingredients of existing products. Developing new food products, similar in appearance to conventional food items, and/or bio-functional foods, whereby risks of chronic disease could be reduced beyond the basic nutritional functionality (*see appendix III - **Bio-Functional-foods***).

Sources of Functional Foods are categorized as naturally derived products and/or industrially synthesized products; naturally occurring functional foods can be subdivided into plant-derived or from animal sources. Functional foods include oats, flaxseeds, cruciferous vegetables, citrus fruits, garlic, tea, grapes, wine, etc. and animal-derived foods include egg, meat, fish, milk, curd, cheese. Industrial products include nutraceuticals and chemically or synthesized or engineered functional foods utilising synthetic biology and nanotechnology. Also, prebiotics and probiotics (or bio-cultures) are of importance to establish or reestablish a functional gut microbiota.

The six main categories of functional foods that have desirable effects towards optimal healthy ageing follow: **Flavonoid, Saponins, Isothiocyanates, Allyl Sulfides, Carotenoids, Catechins.**

Flavonoids

The United States Department of Agriculture has estimated, in the United States adults generally consume **200–250 mg** daily of naturally derived bioflavonoids.

Table 1. shows naturally derived flavonoids: -

Flavonoid	Classification	Dietary sources
Quercetin	flavonols	Vegetables, fruits and beverages, spices
Rutin	flavonols	Green tea, grape seeds, red peppers, apple, citrus fruits, berries, peaches
Macluraxanthone	Xanthones	Hedge apple, dyer's mulberry
Genistein	Isoflavone	fats, oils, beef, red clover, soybeans, psoralea, lupin, fava beans, kudzu
Scopoletin	Coumarin	Vinegar, dandelion coffee
Daidzein	Isoflavone	Soybean, tofu
Taxifolin	flavanonol	Vinegar and citrus fruits
Naringenin	flavanone	grapes
Abyssinones	flavanone	French bean seeds
Rutin	flavonol	apple, citrus fruits, berries, peaches
Eriordictyol	flavanone	Lemon, rose-hips
Fisetin	flavonol	Strawberries, apples, persimmons, onions, cucumbers
Theaflavin	Catechins	Tea leaves, black tea, oolong tea
Poenidin	Anthocyandin	Cranberries, blueberries, plums, grapes, cherries, sweet potatoes
Diosmetin	flavone	vetch
Tricin	flavone	Rice and bran
Biochanin	Isoflavone	Red clover, soya, alfalfa sprouts, peanuts, chickpeas and other legumes

Hesperidin	flavanone	Bitter orange, petit gran, orange, orange juice, lemon and lime
Epicatechin	flavan-3-ol monomers	Milk, chocolate, reduced fat
Myricetin	flavonols	Vegetables, fruits, nuts, berries, tea red wine
Keampferol	flavonols	Apples, grapes, tomatoes, green tea, potatoes, onions, broccoli, Brussel sprouts, squash, cucumbers, lettuce, green beans, peaches, blackberries, raspberries, spinach
Luteolin	flavonols	Celery, broccoli, green peppers, parsley, thyme, dandelion, perilla, chamomile tea, carrots, olive oil, peppermint, rosemary, navel oranges, oregano
Apigenin	flavonols	Milk, chocolate, reduced fat
Resvertrol - flavonols – there are two isomers – cis not		
Polyphenols	Phytoalexin	**Found in stressed plants**
		Red grapes, Japanese knotweed, blueberries, bilberries, cranberries, peanuts, dark chocolate

Chemically, flavonoids are formed of a C_6–C_3–C_6 structure, that consists of two benzene rings linked by a three carbon chains which form an oxygenated heterocyclic carbon ring. The classes of flavonoids, divided in according to their chemical structures: - flavanones, flavones, dihydroflavonols, flavonols, flavan 3-ols, flavanols - including monomers, proanthocyanidins, and other flavanolderived compounds.

Flavonoids are scavengers for radicals (or electrons), and are **anti-inflammatory**, **anti-thrombotic**, help receptor enzyme system and also have inhibitory effects on cyclic-oxygenase and lipoxygenase, and Xanthine oxidase and Aldose reductase inhibitor, flavonoids and non-flavonoid (trans-resveratrol) are also **antioxidants** that help to reduce high levels of undesirable saturated fats and cholesterol in the bloodstream. Flavonoids have benefits of anti-inflammatory protecting cells from oxidative damage (and/or senescence), these dietary antioxidants if combined with the *precursor to NAD+ (nicotinamide adenine dinucleotide)*) are preventive of the development of cardiovascular disease, diabetes, cancer, and cognitive diseases i.e., Alzheimer and dementia via reduction of neurological electron leakage (Garland et le. 2008) and antitumor anti-inflammatory, longevity via activation of **SIRT1** nucleic enzyme (also see appendix, I).

Saponins

Saponins are an important part of functional foods with many health benefits towards optimal healthy ageing. Saponins are steroid, triterpenoid glycosides, common in a large number of plants and plant products. Several biological effects have been ascribed to saponins, research in the membrane, immune stimulant, hypo-cholesterolaemic and anti-carcinogenic properties. These structurally diverse compounds have also been observed to inhibit protozoan also to have the analgesic, anti-nociceptive, antioxidant activity, anti-fungal and antiviral agents. Saponins can form protein complexes with unknown effects when combined with proteins i.e., casein from milk also saponins can disrupt digestion of cholesterol and saturated fats (see Table 2, 3, 4).

Table 2 shows biological activities of saponins:-

Adaptogenic
Adjuvant
Analgesic activity
Antiallergic
Antiedematous
Antiexudative
Antifeedant
Antifungal
Antigenotoxic
Antihepatotoxic inhibitory effect on ethanol absorption
Anti-inflammatory
Antimicrobial
Antimutagenic
Antiobesity
Antioxidant
Antiparasitic
Antiphlogistic
Antiprotozoal
Antipsoriatic
Antipyretic
Antispasmodic
Antithrombotic (effect on blood coagulability)
Antitussive (relieving or preventing cough)
Antiulcer
Antiviral
Chemopreventive
Cytotoxic
Diuretic
Effect on absorption of minerals and vitamins
Effect on animal growth (growth impairment), reproduction
Effect on cognitive behaviour
Effect on ethanol induced amnesia
Effect on morphine/nicotine induced hyperactivity
Effects on ruminal fermentation
Expectorant
Haemolytic
Hepaprotective
Hypocholesterolemic
Hypoglemic
Immunostimulatory effects
Increase permeability of intestinal mucosa cells
Inhibit active nutrient transport
Molluscicidal
Neuroprotective
Reduction in fat absorption
Reduction in ruminal ammonia concentrations
Reductions in stillbirths in swine
Ruminant bloat
Sedative

Hostettmann and Marston, 1995; Lacaille-Dubois and Wagner, 1996; Milgate and Roberts, 1995; Francis et al.,(2002)

Biological Activity of Saponins have been reported to possess a wide range of biological activities, which are summarized and listed alphabetically in Table 2.

While crude isolates, extracts of plants have been utilized in investigations for biological activity, saponins led to the emergence of structure and bio activity relationships (Oda et al., 2000; Gurfinkel and Rao, 2003). The ability of saponins to swell and rupture erythrocytes causing a release of haemoglobin has been investigated for properties of saponins(Oda et al., 2000).

Humans generally do not suffer severe poisoning from saponins, quite the opposite, though toxicity of saponins to insects (insecticidal activity), parasite worms (anthelmintic activity), molluscs (molluscicidal), and fish (piscidal activity) and antifungal, antiviral, and antibacterial activity are well documented (Lacaille-Dubois and Wagner, 1996; Milgate and Roberts, 1995; Francis et al., 2002).

Toxicity of saponins to warm blooded animals is dependent on the method of administration, source, composition, and concentration of the saponin mixture (George, 1965; Oakenfull and Sidhu, 1990). While saponins show toxicity when given intravenously, their toxicity is **much lower when administered orally** which is attributed to low absorption and reduced haemolytic activity in the presence of plasma constituents (Fenwick et al., 1991; George, 1965; Oakenfull and Sidhu, 1990).

A study on the bio availability of soya saponins in humans showed that ingested soya saponins had low absorption rate in human intestinal cells and seem to be metabolized to soya sapogenol B via intestinal microorganisms in vivo and excreted in the faeces (Hu et al., 2004).

Table 3 shows selected plant sources and their constituent saponins

Source	Aglycone	Saponin	Reference
Soybean	Soyasapogenol A	Acetyl soyasaponins A 1 (Ab), A 2 (Af),A 3 ,A 4(Aa), A 5(Ae), A 6,A c,Ad	Yoshiki et al., 1998
	Soyasapogenol B	Soyasaponin DDMP a conjugated I (Bb) βg II (Bc) βa III (Bb) γ g IV (Bc) γ a V (Ba) αg	Yoshiki et al., 1998
	Soyasapogenol E	Soyasaponin Be, Bd	Yoshiki et al., 1998
Chickpea	Soyasapogenol B	DDMP a conjugated saponins	Kerem et al., 2005; Price et al., 1988
Quillaja	Quillaic acid	QS 1-22, S1-12	Kensil and Marciani, 1991; Nord and Kenne, 2000
Horse chestnut	Protoescigenin, barringtogenol C	Aescin (escin): β-aescin, cryptoaescine, α-aescine	World Health Organization, 2001
Alfalfa	Medicagenic acid	I-XV	Oleszek, 1995
	Hederagenin	XVI-XIX	
	Soyasapogenol B	E XX- XXVI	
	Zanhic acid	XXV-XXVI	
Licorice	Glycyrrhetic acid	Glycyrrhizic acid b	World Health Organization, 1999a
Ginseng	20(s)-protopanaxadiol 20(s)-protopanaxatriol	Ra 1–3,Rb 1–3, Rc, Rc2, Rd,Rd2 Re2,Re3, Rf, Rg1,Rg2,Rh1	World Health Organization, 1999
Quinoa	Phytolaccagenic acid Oleanolic acid Hederagenin	Quinoa saponins	Mizui et al., 1990
Oat	Nuategenin	Avenacoside A, B	Onning et al., 1994
Yam (Dioscoera species)	Diosgenin	Dioscin	Hostettmann and Marston, 1995

Fenugreek	Diosgenin, yamogenin, tigogenin, neotigogenin, yuccagenin, lilagenin, gitogenin, neogitogenin, smilagenin, sarsasapoenin	Trigofoenoside Trigonelloside B, C	A-G,	Sauvaire et al., 1995

Key: a is 2,3-dihydro-2,5-dihydroxy-6-methyl-4H-pyran-4-one.
        b is Synonyms: glycyrrhizin, glycyrrhizinic acid.

Table 4 – shows Saponin content of some selected plant material

Source	Saponin content (%)	Reference
Soybean	0.22–0.47	Fenwick et al., 1991
Chickpea	0.23	Fenwick et al., 1991
Green pea	0.18–4.2	Price et al., 1987
Quillaja bark	9–10	San Martin and Briones, 1999
Yucca	10	Oleszek et al., 2001
Fenugreek	4–6	Sauvaire et al., 2000
Alfalfa	0.14–1.71	Fenwick et al., 1991
Licorice root	22.2–32.3	Fenwick et al., 1991
American ginseng (P. quinquefolium L).		
Young leaves	1.42–2.64	Li et al., 1996
Mature leaves	4.14–5.58	Li et al., 1996
Roots (4 year old)	2.44–3.88	Li et al., 1996
Oat	0.1–0.13	Price et al., 1987
Horse chestnut	3–6	Price et al., 1987
Sugar beet leaves	5.8	Price et al., 1987
Quinoa	0.14–2.3	Fenwick et al., 1991

Güçlü Üstündağ, Özlem & Mazza, Giuseppe. (2007). Saponins: Properties, Applications and Processing. Critical reviews in food science and nutrition.

Isothiocyanates

Isothiocyanates are compounds produced by several plants that belong to the **Brassicaceae, Capparaceae** and **Caricaceae** families, such as **Brussel sprouts, garden cress, kale, mustard greens, turnip greens, cabbage, broccoli, watercress, cauliflower horseradish, Japanese radish and cauliflower**, all these vegetables significantly contribute to cancer chemo preventive activity.

Isothiocyanates are rich sources of Sulphur containing compounds called glucosinolates and are a system of physiological defense against pathogen attack. People who consume more than four portions of cruciferous vegetables per week appear to have a lower incidence of diseases (Fahey JW – 2001, Hecht SS et al -2004) These effects appear to be associated with diets rich in fruit and vegetables. Isothiocyanates are the chemical components that occur in cruciferous vegetables that mediate healthy ageing (see table 5 & 6).

Isothiocyanates are derived from the hydrolysis of glucosinolates by the enzyme myrosinase during the conversion of glucosinolates to isothiocyanates. Glucosinolates are thioglycosides that comprise of glycone moiety and a variable glycone-side-chains derived from one of a small number of amino acids. Amino acids accumulate in vegetative members of the Brassicales which include cruciferous vegetables; When plant tissues are damaged or stressed an endogenous plant thioglucosidase, commonly known as myrosinase cleaves the glucosinolate molecule, resulting in the generation of isothiocyanates.

Each glucosinolate forms a different isothiocyanate when hydrolyzed, broccoli is a good source of glucoraphanin. The glucosinolate precursor of sulforaphane. Isothiocyanates are derived from **mustard oil** (2-propenyl-isothiocyanates) and in the herb **wasabi** there is 4-methyl-sulphinylbutyl isothiocyanates (or sulforaphane). And in **Broccoli** - phenethyl-isothiocyanates and in **watercress**; and 3-butenyl-isothiocyanates within **Chinese cabbage (**Wilson et al - 1973) Isothiocyanates conjugate with glutathione leading to induction of oxidative stress and translocation of NRF2 from the cytoplasm to the nucleus and the resultant transcription of **antioxidant** helps gene expression (Fahey JW et al 2012, Verkerk R,et al - 2019)

There is accumulating evidence of isothiocyanatestes impact towards optimal health and healthy ageing and the usage of isothiocyanates towards cancer prevention *(not a cure)*. Moderate quantities of Broccoli, wasabi, Chinese cabbage, Kale and mustard oil *(see table 5 & 6 and appendix I)*.

Table 5 - shows Glucosinolate Content of Selected Cruciferous Vegetables, each glucosinolate forms a different isothiocyanate.

Food (raw)	Serving	Total Glucosinolates (mg)
Brussels sprouts	½ cup (44 g)	104
Garden cress	½ cup (25 g)	98
Mustard greens	½ cup, chopped (28 g)	79
Turnip	½ cup, cubes (65 g)	60
Cabbage, savoy	½ cup, chopped (45 g)	35
Kale	1 cup, chopped (67 g)	67
Watercress	1 cup, chopped (34 g)	32
Kohlrabi	½ cup, chopped (67 g)	31
Cabbage, red	½ cup, chopped (45 g)	29
Broccoli	½ cup, chopped (44 g)	27
Horseradish	1 tablespoon (15 g)	24
Cauliflower	½ cup, chopped (50 g)	22
Bok choy (pak choi)	½ cup, chopped (35 g)	19

Table 6 - shows functional food sources of selected Isothiocyanates and their Glucosinolate Precursors: -

Isothiocyanate	Glucosinolate (precursor)	Food Sources
Allyl isothiocyanate	Sinigrin	Broccoli, Brussels sprouts, cabbage, horseradish, kohlrabi, mustard, radish
Benzyl isothiocyanate	Glucotropaeolin	Cabbage, garden cress, Indian cress
Phenethyl isothiocyanate	Gluconasturtiin	Watercress

Sulforaphane	Glucoraphanin	Broccoli, Brussels sprouts, cabbage, cauliflower, kale

Isothiocyanate epigenetic regulation, the deacetylation of histones by HDAC restricts access of transcription factors to the DNA that suppresses transcription, can potentially promote differentiation and apoptosis in transformed (precancerous) cells; Isothiocyanates inhibit HDAC expression and activity in cultured cancer cells   HDAC activity was reduced in blood cells following ingestion of 68g (one cup) of sulforaphane-rich broccoli sprouts (see Table 5). Isothiocyanates may also affect microRNA-mediated gene silencing though further research is necessary *(Abbaoui B et al – 2017)*.

Allyl Sulfides

Organosulfur (allyl sulfides) compounds found in allium vegetables such as **garlic and onions** which are known anti-carcinogenic agents. Allyl sulfides increase the production of glutathione S-transferase

Garlic also contain phytochemicals (especially if stressed), such as quercetin and allyl sulfides, which are linked to cardiovascular health, immunity function ..., also total white blood cell count has been enhanced significantly with moderate intake of garlic.

Allyl sulfides are more powerful inducers than the methyl or propyl derivatives, and within the allyl series, the disulfide is a more potent inducer than the monosulfide. Thiosulfonates are allylsulfide compounds including allicin, diallyldisulfide (DADs), diallyl sulfide (DAS), diallyl trisulfide, Sallylmercaptocysteine, S-allylcysteineallyl and methyl sulfide (see figure 1b & 1c)

Garlic derived DADS and DATS influenced anaerobic cysteine metabolism, elevating the activity of enzymes involved in the normal kidneys. DATS inhibits ALDH activity in the kidneys, showing a new pharmacological property of garlic derived allyl trisulfide. ALDH inhibition can lead to an increase concentration of aldehydes, the toxicity of which could be used in the reduction of senescent cells.

Garlic-derived allyl sulfides relates to sulfane Sulphur metabolism or with ALDH activity though further studies are required. Garlic-derived allyl sulfides and enzymes involved with the synthesis and biodegradation of H_2S again further research on catalytic activity, and protein antibody level, and on gene expression is required; Allyl sulfides make alterations in cholesterol, arachidonic acid, phospholipids and thiols account for changes in membrane functionality. Allyl sulfides are recognized for ability to suppress cellular proliferation by the induction of apoptosis *(see figure 1b & 1c and Appendix I).*

Allyl sulfides derived from garlic have the ability of to suppress tumor proliferation both in vitro and in vivo. This anti-neoplastic effect is greater for lipid-soluble than water-soluble, concentration and duration of exposure will increase effects of lipid- and water solubility, may relate to an increase in membrane fluidity and suppression of integrin glycoprotein mediated adhesion. This increased histone acetylation, increased intracellular calcium and elevated cellular peroxide production. The composition of the entire diet and epigenetic factors will possibly determine the true future benefits that perhaps will arise from allyl Sulphur compounds from garlic and other genus Allium functional foods.

Carotenoids

Carotenoids have important physiological actions known is the provitamin A activity, Vitamin A is essential for normal vision, gene expression, embryonic development, immunological functions and control of metabolic processes.

Table 7 shows examples of functional food that includes Carotenoids: -

β-carotene
Brussel sprouts, Karat bananas, peaches, pepper (red, orange, green), west Indian cherry, apricot, broccoli, buriti, carrots, gac oil, kale, mango, red palm oil, spinach, sweet potato, tomatoes
β-cryptoxanthin
Persimmon and pitanga
Lutein
Broccoli, green leafy vegetables, yellow and green peppers
Zeaxanthin
Buriti, Chinese wolfberry and orange and red peppers
Lycopene
Carrots, guava, tomatoes and watermelon

Carotenoids are especially abundant in yellow-orange fruits and vegetables and in dark green, leafy vegetables. Though carotenoids are also found in animal derived products e.g., dairy products, eggs, some fish and seafood.

Vitamin A is an important micronutrient within functional foods as carotenoids are mainly present in plants. Provitamin A activity exerted by some carotenoids, influences diverse molecular and cellular processes, involved in risk reduction of several chronic diseases; these are certain types of cancers, cardiovascular disease, type 2 diabetes, age-related macular degeneration and cataracts and other diseases.

Catechins

Table 8 shows the composition of major components in <u>green tea</u>, Catechins are also found in other products i.e., wine, tea, cacao, coffee, and wild berries raspberries and acai berries.

Components	% of Dry weight
Catechins	30
Theanine	3
Amino acids	4
Caffeine	3
Carbohydrates	11
Proteins	15
Organic acids	2
Lipids	3
Minerals	10
Chlorophyll and other pigments	0.5

Green Tea - comprises of a verity of soluble substances i.e. catechins, caffeine, theanine, chlorophyll, organic acids, and vitamins as shown in Table 8. Notice there is a large quantity of Catechins in green tea, in comparison to other soluble substances green tea has more catechins compared to other teas such as black tea or oolong tea, tea. Catechins and polyphenols are effective scavengers of reactive oxygen species in vitro which function as antioxidants that form flavonoids of which has a protective function from free radicals. For this rational detox Teas incorporate large amounts of catechins that assist with weight loss efforts by increasing physiological magnitude of energy by utilising stored body fat for energy towards optimal healthy ageing.

Probiotics

Probiotics are bacterial species and metabolites found in functional foods, the microbiota are found in the lungs, stomach, intestinal tract and colon.

This list of probiotics is rudimentary:

Bifildobacterium lactis	Lactobacillus paracasei
Enterococcus faecium	Lactobacillus salivarius
Lactobacillus acidophilus	Lactobacillus bulgaricus
Lactobacillus plantarum	Bacillus coagluans
Lactococcus lactis	Bifildobacterium breve
Lactobacillus rhamnsus	Bifildobacterium lungum …

The above probiotics (or bio-cultures) are an important part of immunity and have a reconstruction effect in the gut, also assists in cellular metabolism and blood calcium levels and bile metabolism, also the synthesis of vitamins. This improves immunity, and the nerve system, and endocrine system and enhancement of glycemic control; all of which effect the epigenetics in a positive way *(Tonucci LB et al - 2017)* towards optimal healthy ageing. Similar probiotics are incorporated into foods i.e., bioyogurt and fermented milk, cheese, and fruit-based drinks. Probiotic mechanisms include colonization of host-tissues in the gastrointestinal tract, improve glucose metabolism, improve skin, stomach, colon to create a healthy microbiota. The mechanism of gut microbiota ameliorates intestinal wall permeability for healthier mineral absorption providing fibrous prebiotics is also included *(see functional foods and Bio-Functional-foods letter within appendix III)*

Nanotechnology

Nanotechnology engineering will produce effective nanoscale nutrient carriers of functional foods, thereby nanoparticles are utilized for developing foods with higher nutritional value, sensory response, process-ability, and shelf life. These various types of particles will enable molecular suiting and delivery system for specific physiological needs. Applied nanotechnology will improve the functionality of functional foods to provide physiological benefits; prepared via fortification with vitamins and minerals more than mandatory requirements with additional bioactive ingredients and enhancement via epigenetic modifications and selectively breeding and engineering via synthetic biology of various plant and bacteria species... Functional foods maybe, emulsions, and foams that exhibit complexity and diversity though with natural appearance.

Application of nanotechnology in food science utilizing a delivery system for encapsulating, protecting, and controlling the release of micronutrients via functional foods towards optimal health with benefits to reduce the risk of chronic diseases. Examples of nutraceuticals are natural foods, including antioxidants, dietary supplements, fortified dairy products, and citrus fruits, and vitamins, minerals, herbals, milk, and cereals.

Future functional foods will be nanoparticles that are biological molecules found naturally in certain foods that provide physiological benefits thereby diminishing the risks of many diseases. The reduced particle size that nanotechnology provides improve properties of biological molecules, improvement of delivery, solubility, prolonged gastrointestinal time, and efficient cellular absorption

The majority of functional food nanoparticles conventionally were the colloid group (i.e., co-enzymes); the stabilization of colloidal particles is achieved via adsorbing surfactants and polymers and by coating the nanoparticles with chemically bonding molecules.

Micro emulsions are thermodynamically stable systems, formed spontaneously when surfactants and other biological components are added to water under the right environmental conditions. Generally, the new functional bioactive foods consist of micronutrients inside nanoparticles. Utilizing surfactants, lipids and carbohydrates; all compacted in a small particle size of < 500 nm. These new functional foods will include improved bioavailability, centrifugal separation, greater stability, and higher optical clarity (Momin et al., 2013; Joye et al., 2014; Sekhon, 2010).

Nutriments are often lost during processing or storage of food because of the enzymatically unstable nature of many of the micronutrients that are incorporated into food products The stability of micronutrients is important and a successful delivery system would incorporate micronutrients within functional foods while release in the bioactive form upon consumption of food for digestion.

The design and production of food-grade nanoparticles that food manufacturers may utilize to develop effective micronutrient is a potential resource for encapsulating and enhancement and stability, functionality, and bioavailability of micronutrients for functional foods and food packaging. Several applications of nanotechnologies have become apparent with usage of nanoparticles, such as liposomes, nano-emulsions, biopolymeric nanoparticles, and cubosomes, as well as the development of **nano-sensors**, with the objective of ensuring food safety **Nasr, Nasr.** (2015)

Lipid-based nano-encapsulation systems boost antioxidant performance, enhancing solubility and bioavailability for manufactures the principal lipid-based nano-encapsulation systems with potential use in food and nutraceutical industries. Thus, nanotechnology offers food technologists new opportunities to innovate in encapsulation and controlled release of food materials, as well as providing enhanced bioavailability, stability, and shelf life for sensitive ingredients (Mozafari et al., 2012). Nano-encapsulation packaging is advantageous in developing designer probiotic bacterial preparations with the potential for locating gastrointestinal tract where the probiotics/bio-cultures interact with specific receptors. The health-enhancing properties of polyphenols have attracted much attention in recent years. A milk-based protein has been used to prepare oil-in-water, sodium caseinate stabilized nano-emulsions. The immobilization of fat droplets, composed of high melting temperature milk fat triglycerides, has provided protection against packaged nutrient degradation and enhance food flavor and texture, to reduce fat content, or to encapsulate nutrients, such as vitamins, and increase functionality and stability (*Wai-Yee Fung, Kay-Hay Yuen, and Min-Tze Liong - 2011*).

Reference: Earl R, Thomas PR (eds) (1994) **Opportunities in the nutrition and food sciences: research challenges and the next generation of investigators**. National Academies Press Fahey JW, Wehage SL, Holtzclaw WD, et al. **Protection of humans by plant glucosinolates: efficiency of conversion of glucosinolates to isothiocyanates by the gastrointestinal microflora**. Cancer Prev Res (Phila). 2012;5(4):603-611.Fahey JW, Zalcmann AT, Talalay P. **The chemical diversity and distribution of glucosinolates and isothiocyanates among plants**. Phytochemistry. 2001;56(1):5-51German, E, et el., **Hepatic metabolism of Diallyl Disulfide in rat and man.** Xenobiotica, 2003. 33(12) pp 1185-99Gould BS. **Collagen formation and fibogenesis with special reference to the role of ascorbic acid**. International Review of Cytology. 1963:15:301-361.Hecht SS. **Chemoprevention by Isothiocyanates. In:** Kelloff GJ, Hawk ET, Sigman CC, eds. Promising Cancer Chemo preventive Agents, Volume 1: Cancer Chemo preventive Agents Totowa, NJ: Humana Press; 2004:21-35. Hogue, D.E., **vitamin E, selenium and other factors related to muscular dystrophy in limbs.** Cornell nutrition conference for feed manufacturers proceedings, 1958: pp32-9. Khattak M. **Biological significance of ascorbic acid (vitamin C) in human health**- A review Pakistan Journal of Nutrition. 2004:3:5-13

Knowles HJ, Ravel RR, Harris AL el al. **Effects of ascorbate on the activity of hypoxa-inducable factor in cancer cells**. Cancer Research. 2003:63:1764-1764.Li, P.et al. p27(Kipl) **stabilisation and G(1) arrest by 1,25-dihydroxyvitamin D(3) in ovarian cancer cells mediated though down-regulation of cyclin E/ cyclindependent kinase 2 and skp1-cullin-F-box protein/skp2 ubiquitin ligase.** J, Biol Chem 279, 2526025267 (2004) Piyathilake CJ, Bell WC, Johanning GL et al. **The accumulation of ascorbic acid by squamous cell carcinomas of the lung and larynx is associated globe methylation of DNA**. Cancer. 2000:98:171-176. Sharma, R.A.A.J. Gescher and W.P.Steward, **Curcumin: The story of far.** Eur J Cancer 2005. 41(13): pp1955-68Thakur, vs.., k. Gupta, **Green Tea polyphenols cause cell cyclic arrest and apoptosis in prostate cancer by suppressing in class 1 histone deacetylases** carsinogenesis, 2012. 33(2): pp. 377-84Tonucci LB., Olbrirch Dos Santos KM., Licursi de Oliveerirra L., Rocha Ribeiro SM., Duarte Martino HS. **Clinical applications of probiotics in type 2 diabetes mellitus: a ramderized, double-blind, placebo-controlled study**. Clin Nutr 2017;36(1):85-92Traber HG, Stevens JF, **Vitamin C and E: beneficial effects on mechanistic perspective**. Free Radical Biology and Medicine. 201151:1000-1013.udali S, Guarini P, Morrozzi S, Choi SW, Friso S. **Cardiovascular epigenetics: from DNA methylation to microRNAs.** Mol Aspect. Med 2013:883-901Thomson C, Bloch AS, Hasler CM, Kubena K, Earl R, Heins J. (1999) **Position of the American dietetic association.** J.Am Diet Assoc 99(10):1278–1285Van Robertson wb, Schwartz B. Ascorbic **acid and the formation of collagen**, the journal of Biological Chemistry. 953:201:689-696.

29/04/21

Weststrate JA, Van Poppel G, Verschuren PM (2002) **Functional foods, trends and future.** Br J. Nutr 88(S2):S233–S235Wilson CWM, Loh HS. **Vitamin C and colds** The Lancet. 1973:3:5-13. Verkerk R, Schreiner M, Krumbein A, et al. **Glucosinolates in Brassica vegetables: the influence of the food supply chain on intake, bioavailability and human health.** Mol Nutr Food Res. 2009;53 Suppl 2: S219.Zhang Y. **Cancer-preventive isothiocyanates: measurement of human exposure and mechanism of action**. Mutat Res. 2004;555(1-2):173-190.

Chapter 2

A brief introduction to Epigenetics

Nutriepigenomics reveal how diet determine *epigenetic modifications both histone and Non-coding RNAs of the human genome regulating both to health and disease.* Histone modifications is the mechanism by which methylation and acetylation of histone tails regulates the epigenetic cellular system.

Each of the eight histone proteins make an octamer (see figure 1a & 1b), and a combination of post-translational modifications (methylation and acetylation) occur at sites on the nucleosol histone-core tails. Although other modifications occur, phosphorylation, Sumoylation, ubiquitylation(Ub), GlcNAcylation, citrullination, krotonilation, and isomerization. The later three are more recent discoveries, these modifications add or remove from histone amino acid residues via a set of enzymatic reactions.

Post-translational modifications (PTMs) of histone-tails have resultant changes in chromatin that may induce and increase or decrease in DNA-histone affinity (*udali S, Guarini et al - 2013*) an increase of DNA-histone affinity results in transcriptional repression the opposite results with relaxation of the DNA coils around the histone proteins for gene expression. Histone methylation *normally is on arginine, lysine, and histone residues; the magnitude and location determines transcriptional activation or repression of gene expression (see figure 1a & 1b).*

Figure 1a shows a graphical representation of the structural chromosomal *chromatin with coiled DNA, the nucleosol DNA coils around the histone proteins to make a nucleosome that coil to make a chromatin fiber that coils to make a chromosome.*

Figure 1a - the DNA coils around the octamer/nucleosome core complexes which are bound firmly with DNA for gene repression.

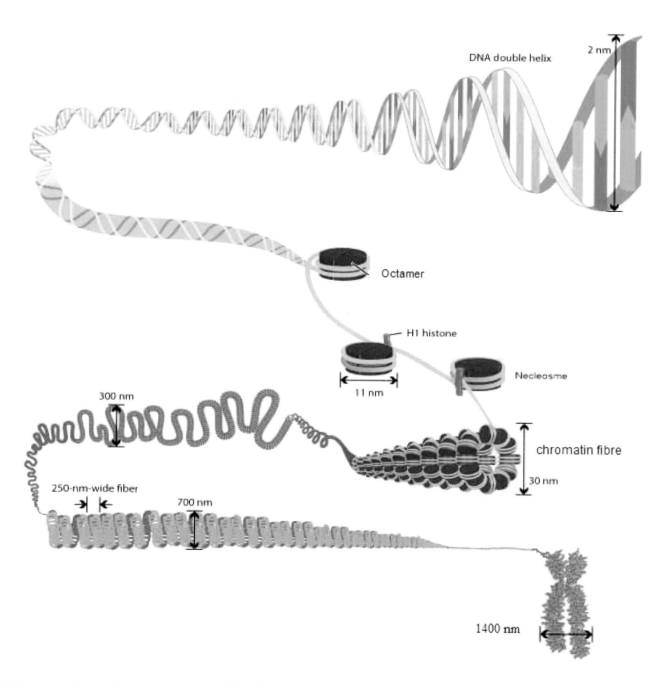

Figure 1a shows a graphical representation of the structural chromosomal chromatin with coiled DNA, the nucleosol DNA coils around the histone proteins to make a nucleosome that coils to make a chromatin fiber that coils to make a chromosome.

The process of Acetylation unbinds the DNA loosely around the octamer so that gene expression can occur, the chromatin fiber consists of DNA wound around histone protein complexes that is the nucleosome coiled into the hairpin structure chromatin fiber; acetylation of histones effect how accessible the DNA is for repression or expression, that is for gene expression (see figure 1b).

Histone modifications

Histone modifications HTMs are diverse, including phosphorylation, methylation, acetylation, ubiquitylation and during meiotic spermatogenic cell division most haploid genome are misplaced by protamine, though not all some are retained so to transmit genetic information to the progeny. However, histone modifications are implicated with cell senescence, cancer, cardiovascular disease, obesity diabetes and many other epigenetic modifications.

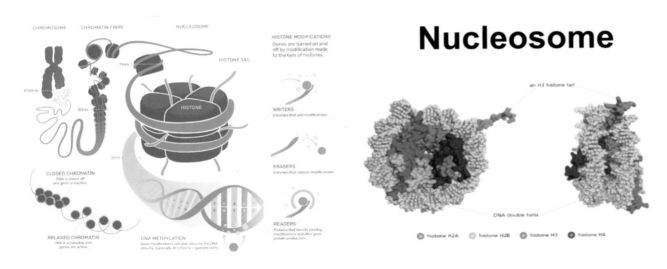

Figure 1b shows graphical representation and x-ray diffraction analysis (front and side orientation) of the nucleosome and histone tails providing access for transcription, mostly controlled by histone proteins. the nucleosome consists of an octamer made of <u>two</u> **subunits** contain four histone proteins: **H2A**, **H2B**, **H3**, and **H4**. (With tails) that is a total of eight histone proteins, 2 tetramers (H2-H4) and 2 (H2A-H2B) dimers in the histone/octamer core complex. The ammo acid linker proteins – H1 etc.... functions to bind and stabilize inter-nucleosol DNA, the linker DNA joins octamer together to make the nucleosome; the histone proteins undergo post-translational (PTM) and post transcriptional modifications in different ways (some are salt dependent). Some histone modifications disrupt nucleosol DNA interactions, thereby the nucleosomes **unwind** or relax for gene expression.

Histone *methylation* can activate or suppress gene *expression in accordance to different lysine dependent states (i.e. Mono-methyl, Di-methyl, or Tri-methyl states; the demethylated function is in reverse (relaxes the DNA coils) on the histone-tails during transcription. There are* **seven** *transcriptional regulatory core histone modifications on the H3 histone-tail that is:– 2 active promoters* (**H3K9ac**, **H3K4me3**), 2 enhancer promoters (**H3K4me1** (stem cell line), **H3K27ac**), 1 transcribed gene bodies (**H3K36me3**), 1 polycomb promoters (**H3K27me3**), 1 hetero*chromatin* (**H3K9me3**) it is possible to define *chromatin profile status (biomarkers) of the genome via the histone-tail modification epigenetic biomarker status (see figure, 1d & Appendix, I, II).*

Other than **Acetylation(Ac) and methylation(Me)** there are other types of histone modifications have been discovered:- **phosphorylation(P), sumoylation, ubiquitylation(Ub), GlcNAcylation, citrullination, krotonilation, and isomerization** the later three are more recent discoveries, all the above modifications **add or remove from histone protein's amino acid residues** via a set of enzymatic reactions *(see figure 1c & 1d, and Appendix, I, II).*

Histone proteins are (H1-linker protein, H3, H4, H2A, H2B) which are dependent on Post-Translational Modification (PTMs); PTMs normally are reversible and effect all chromatin remodeling and centromere formation. PMTs are classified as reader, writer and eraser and are either: Effectors(enhancers) or Presenters(promoters). Histone PTMs may alter the chromatin state making it active, inactive or poised state. PTM associations may occur with cis or trans events on same or nearby histone tails, within the same or neighboring nucleosome *(Zang T et al – 2015).*

Histone Protein Tails

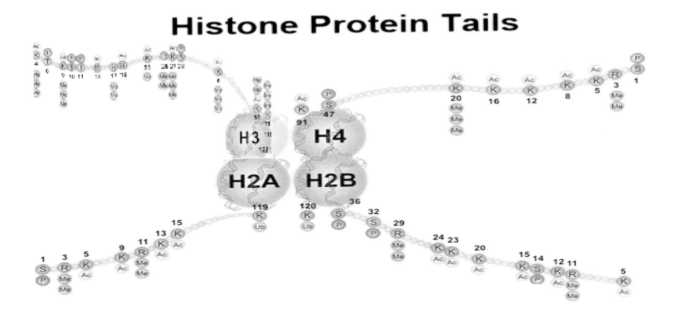

Figure 1c - *shows adapted graphical representation* showing numbered *Histone modifications with Histone-tails, showing the modifications are transactional epigenetic markers that undergo events via: Acetylation(**Ac**), methylation(**Me**), Phosphorylation(**P**), ubiquitylation(**Ub**)* all are necessary to allow activity of the chromatin remodeling complex.

Methylation activates or represses gene *expression depending on which residue is methylated; Methylation of histone methyltransferases (HMTs), of Lysine SET domain containing (histone tails) and Non-SET domain containing histone cores. All of the above modifications* **add or remove** from *histone proteins amino acid residues via a set of enzymatic reactions (see figure 1c & 1d, appendix, I, II)*

Mechanisms of nutrition on epigenetics

Three epigenetic mechanisms: **DNA methylation**, **histone modification**, and **non-coding RNA** that is involved in gene silencing.

The nutritional variables that effect the function of the epigenome are biological molecules of vitamins, minerals and herbs that have epigenetic benefit diminishing the onset of illness; achieved via epigenetic enhancement during **histone acetylation** of the HAT enzymes occurs on the ε-amino lysine residue. Histone acetyltransferase (**HAT**) **inhibits gene expression**, and the HDAC enzyme, histone deacetylase (**HDAC) enables gene expression**. Thus, HAT and HDAC are involved in control gene expression switching gene expression <u>off</u> (methyl- groups) or <u>on</u> (acetyl- groups) via structural histones and histone-tails that compress the DNA for repression and uncoil the DNA for gene expression. HAT and HDAC are reversible epigenetic modifications that nutritional molecules are effectors. Each histone octamer is wrapped by 147 bp of DNA to form a nucleosome, the spacing between each base-pair (bp) varies between 30 and 100 and can be modified by nucleosome repositioning complexes. Figure 1d (also see figure 1a, 1b & 1c) shows HAT & HDAC reversible histone modifications that are dependent biological molecules. Ref:(2013). Acetyltransferases (HAT) for Neurological Therapeutics. Neurotherapeutics: the journal of the American Society for Experimental Neuro Therapeutics)

DNA methylation

DNA methylation regulates gene expression via the addition of a methyl group on the 5' position on the pyrimidine ring of the nucleotide, this methylation occurs on the amino acid cytosine flanked by a guanine that yields a 5'-cytosinephosphate-guanine-3'(CpG) methylation.   Also, methylation occurs on the cytosine neighboring other nucleotides for non-CpG methylation.

Approximately 5% of cytosines are methylated at the global level, with hypermethylation observed in areas of hetero-chromatin and hypo-methylation. High densities of CpG sites are localized to repetitive DNA, specifically the localization of methyl-cytosines in relation to the gene and the density of CpG islands.

DNA methylation occurs at CpG sites though most of the genome is CpG poor, there are segments of 300-3000 bp with a 65% observed to expected ratio of CpG sites that are called CpG islands (CGIs). The CpG islands are localized to the promoter region of 70% of human genes, including tissue-specific genes, and developmentally regulated genes vital for stem cells due to distinctive topology that is reprogrammed with the gametes. DNA methylation is regulated via DNA methyltransferases (DNMT) there is DNMT 1, DNMT 3a, DNMT 3b though DNMT 1 is predominant in humans *(Duygu et al 2013 - also see Appendix, I, II).*

DNA *methylation* function is to transfer a methyl group (CH3–) to 5' end of the *DNA (cytosine) sequence via DNMTs and S-adenosyl methionine (SAM) as the methyl group donor, cytosine is adjoining to the guanine residue refired to as CpG inland.* Gene sequencing is enriched at CpG and if present in the gene promoter region transcriptional *repression will occur, however if present on the exon region transcriptional activation will occur (udali S, Guarini - 2013, Mazzio EA et al – 2012).*

DNA demethylation

There are various pathways for **DNA demethylation** and the **passive** removal of a methyl group (CH3) of 5-mC, during de-methylation 5-mC is demethylated for cellular division during mitosis for replication; however **active** de-methylation occurs with **non-replicating neurons. DNA demethylation** is the process of removal of a methyl group from cytosines. **DNA demethylation can** be passive or active. The passive process takes place in the absence of methylation of newly synthesized **DNA** strands by DNMT1 during several replication cycles.

DNA Hydroxy methylation

The ten-eleven transferase (TET) enzyme catalyzes an oxidation reaction that converts 5-methylcytosinein to 5-hydroxymethylcytosine before subsequent steps that ultimately yield an unmodified cytosine (see figure 1f). Regions of hydroxy methylated DNA are considered to be sites of active demethylation and have been associated with an increase in gene expression *(Tammen et al., 2015)*. In the presence of a hydroxy-methyl group on the 5 position of cytosine in CpG dinucleotides is a biomarker, considered a transient step in active demethylation of DNA.

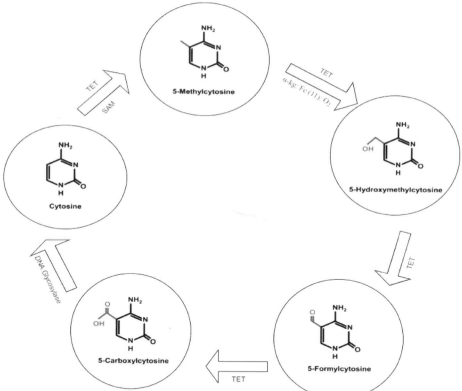

Figure 1f - shows - proposed mechanism of active demethylation by ten-eleven transferase (TET). The enzyme TET acts on a methylated cytosine to catalyze a series of reactions to yield transitions to hydroxy methyl cytosine, formyl methyl cytosine, and carboxyl cytosine. The enzyme DNA glycosylase catalyzes the final step to yield an unmethylated cytosine. DNMT, DNA methyltransferase; SAM, S-adenosylmethionine. (Tammen, S.A., Friso, S., Choi, S.W., 2013.

Epigenetics: the link between nature and nurture. Mol Asp Med 34(4), 753e764), see Glossary.

RNA modifications

Non-coding *RNAs are small nucleolar RNAs, ribosomal RNAs, long regulatory non-coding RNAs(lncRNAs), microRNAs, small interfering RNAs(siRNAs) and piwi-interacting(piRNAs) RNAs and other regulatory RNAs involved in functional tissue specificity that are nucleic* **transcriptional and intergenerational signaling for inheritable *phenotype*.** The micro*RNAs are transcribed and folded into a hairpin structure and cleaved via a DROSHA complex the resultant hairpin precursor pre-miRNA is transported from the nucleus to the cytoplasm via exportin-5 and unites with a Dicer complex to become a mature microRNA. A* negative regulatory RNA-inducing silencing complex (RISC) results with degradation of the mRNA sequence, thus regulating protein synthesis; also important in post transcriptional regulation of many diseases. Micro*RNAs can be utilized as epigenetic biomarkers for various cancer types (Earl R, Thomas PR (1994), Duygu B et al - 2013, Wong NW et al-2017, Chatterjee et al - 2013).*

Environmental factors can remodel *epigenomic somatic tissues and sperm of which is dynamic and vulnerable to internal and external environmental changes. During spermatogenesis DNA modifications are erased, reconstructed and the histones are replaced via arginine-rich protamine in the sperm. The fundamental* question of how parental diet and lifestyle alter epigenetic *phenotype* and perhaps behavior, other mechanistic signals transfer environmental and epigenetic fluctuations.

Table 10 shows the types, and Characteristics, and Major Functions of RNA.				
RNA	Abundance	Size (nt)	Stability	Function
mRNA	2%-5% of total	1000-1500	Unstable to very stable	Carries the genetic information
NON-CODING RNAS (NCRNAS)				
Short ncRNAs				

miRNAs	<1% of total	19-031	Stable to very stable	Regulation of proliferation, differentiation, and apoptosis
siRNAs	<1% of total			Post-transcriptional gene silencing
RNAs	<1% of total			mRNA splicing
tRNAs	15% of total			Decode a mRNA sequence into a protein
circRNAs	5%-10% of total	>50		Protein production and transporting miRNAs inside the cell/Regulation of mRNA splicing - Chen (2016)
Long ncRNAs				
rRNA	80.00%	>200	Very stable	Essential for protein synthesis

Mitochondrial DNA methylation

Mitochondria is the control center for lipid (fat) metabolism, the Mitochondria DNA (mtDNA) is a 16,569 base-pair though mtDNA is absent of histones and comprised of a H (heavy) and L (light) DNA strand that encodes for 37 genes: 13 oxidative phosphorylation related protein-encoding genes, 22 transfer RNAs and 2 ribosomal RNAs mtDNA is said to modify 5-mC and 5-hmC though these epigenetic modifications are still debatable, these are regulative of skeletal and heart muscles, more non-CpG (than CpG) is methylated in the Dloop region of the circular mrDNA leading to activation of ND1 and repression of ND6, mtDNA has dependence of: mitochondrial transcription factor 2, mitochondrial transcription factor A and mitochondrial RNA polymerase. The rate of lipid or fat metabolism is regulated via mtDNA that is encoded on the X chromosome inherited on the maternal side, if the maternal is showing obesity, the slow metabolic biomarkers are not always expressed if the recipient is in acknowledgement of functional foods and participates in regular physical exercise. (Also see future of *epigenetics and Bio-functional-foods*)

Histone *acetylation*

Histone *acetylation* (Ac) occurs on the ε-amino lysine residue and promotes *DNA unfolding – CoA (acetyl coenzyme A) and lysine where HAT (histone acetyltransferase enzyme, inhibits gene expression - i.e., repression for immunological defense) and HDAC (histone deacetylase enzyme, HDAC enables nucleic gene expression), n-butyrate is a HDAC inhibitor where HATs are co-activators during transcription.   HATs categories are: GCN5, MYST(MOZ), P300/CBP and SRC/p160 of the nuclear receptor co-activator family. Histone and non-histone proteins are catalyzed via HATs. Reversible histone acetylation catalyzed via HATs and HDATs also histone acetylation can inhibit H1-mediated salt insolubility assisting salt solubility concentrations that effects binding and relaxation of DNA coils on the hairpin nucleosome structure. Thus, HATS and HDAC are involved in the control gene expression switching gene expression off or on.   This effect is consistent with the expected large reduction in electron density on the amino nitrogen upon acetylation thus, making coordination with the coenzyme copper much less strong; the structure of histones shows the patterns of histone acetylation and methylation are quite precise and important mechanisms for epigenetic alteration of gene expression (See figure 1c & 1d and appendix, I)*

Histone *methylation*

Histone *methylation* (Me) causes local formation of **hetero**chromatin, which is reversible also can activate or suppress gene *expression in accordance to different lysine dependent states (i.e. Mono-methyl, Di-methyl, or Tri-methyl (binds) states;* The de-methylated function is in reverse (relaxes) the *histone-tails during transcription. There are* **seven** transcriptional regulatory core *histone modifications on the 3 histone-tail that is:–* two active promoters (**H3K9ac**, **H3K4me3**), two enhancer promoters (**H3K4me1** (stem cell line), **H3K27ac**), one transcribed gene bodies (**H3K36me3**), one polycomb promoters(**H3K27me3**), one heterochromatin (**H3K9me3**) it is possible to define *chromatin profile states of the genome via the seven histone-tail modification marker stats (figure 1d, table 10 and see Appendix, I, II).*

Table 11 shows Epigenetic Marks and Their Effect on Gene Expression.

Epigenetic mark	Description	Effect on gene expression	Notes
DNA methylation	Addition of methyl group to 50 position on pyrimidine ring of cytosine	Decrease expression	Effect depends on genomic context. Promoter-associated CpG islands are rarely methylated where as methylation at CpG Island shores is more variable and inversely associated with gene expression.
DNA hydroxymethylation	Placement of hydroxymethyl group on 50 position of pyrimidine ring of cytosine	Increase expression	Considered to be a transient mark in the active demethylation process.
H3K27ac	Acetylation of lysine 27 on histone 3	Increase expression	Associated with transcriptional initiation in euchromatin.
H3K9ac	Acetylation of lysine 9 on histone 3	Increase expression	Associated With transcriptional initiation in euchromatin.
H4K16ac	Acetylation of lysine 16 on histone 4	Increase expression	Localized to active genes and enhancer regions.
H3K27me3	Trimethylation of lysine 27 on histone 3	Decrease	Associated with gene repression of inactive developmental loci, placed by polycombrep repressive complex.
H3K36me3	Trimethylation of lysine 36 on histone 3	Increase expression	Co-localizes with RNA polymerase II during elongation.
H3K4me1/me2/me3	Mono/di/trimethylation of lysine4 on histone 3	Increase expression	During active transcription.
H3K9me3	Trimethylation of lysine 9 on histone 3	Decrease expression	Associated with repressive heterochromatin
H3K9me1	Monomethylation oflysine 9 on histone 3	Increase expression	Associated with accessible chromatin during active transcription.
H4K20me1	Monomethylation oflysine 20 on histone 4	Increase expression	Associated with accessible chromatin during active transcription, catalyzed by PR-Set 7.

H2AK119Ub1	Monoubiquitination of lysine 119 on histone 2		A Decrease Catalyzed by Bmi1subunit of polycomb repressive complex 1.II.

Nutritional effects of functional foods on epigenetic activities

Functional foods are bioactive and help to prevent degenerative conditions such as Alzheimer disease, molecular degenerative disease, encephalopathy, arthritis... (list is exhausting) are internal physiological factors that affect genetic(indirectly) and directly epigenetic modifications; caused by the onset of cell senescence/ageing, though effect can be reduced in favor of healthy ageing with appropriate nutrition. Functional foods and Bio-functional-foods also incorporates all micronutrients and microfauna and microflora know as **microbiota**. Microbiota may be derived from fibrous nutrients together with probiotics in bioyogurt, algae and other functional foods. with adequate fibrosus nutrition, obesity related metabolic diseases may be reduced via the HDAC biological dependent pathways via repression or expression of genes (see figure 1d, and appendixes).

Providing nutritional intake is adequate, Vitamins, minerals, herbal supplements and micronutrients within functional foods will enhance epigenetic modifications and immunity shall function with reduction of toxins and oxidants, i.e. vitamins A, D and green tea are good examples of antioxidants. The nutritional benefits of fresh and functional foods containing multi vitamins, minerals and herbs are beneficial towards optimal health and healthy ageing. Essential Vitamins A, B2, B6, B9, B12, C, D, E, K... and selenium dependent glutathione and other antioxidants i.e... Trans-Resveratrol also the precursor NAD+, sirtuins and other enhancing nutrients together with bio-cultures will assist towards optimal healthy ageing.

Vitamin C is not produced in-vitro to the physiology therefore daily consumption is important. Vitamin C assist with the regulation of collagen synthesis and essential in bone formation, maintenance of healthy gums, and wound healing there has been suggestions for vitamin C treatment as preventative usage for: influenza, upper respiratory tract infections, diabetes, cataracts, glaucoma, macular degeneration, atherosclerosis, stroke, heart disease and even cancer

(Traber et al 2011) vitamin C is noted as a co-factor for histone modifications and reduces oxidative stress and also is neuro-protective and cancer chemo preventative *(Li, P.et al – 2004)*.

Polyunsaturated fats are healthy - unsaturated fats and saturated fats refer to the quantity of hydrogen within the lipid structure of the fat, saturated fats comprise of many hydrogen bonds that are less healthy than unsaturated referred to as polyunsaturated fats that are Omiga-3 fatty acids and omiga-6 fatty acids (see table 11). A high fat diet of saturated animal derived fats **changes histone-tail modifications in unwanted ways at the gluconeogenic gene loci**; Were as the he healthier **Omiga-3 polyunsaturated fats intake has a stabilizing effect. Omiga-3 fatty acids are** found in Flaxseed oil, evening primrose oil and fish oil that increase D3, D5 and D6 desaturase enzyme activities that have a healthy dietary effect on blood platelets and immunity.

Table 11 shows the difference between omaga-3 and omega-6 fatty acids derived from functional foods:	
omega-3 fatty acids	
Alpha-linoenic acid	Wild fruit, berries, leafy vegetables, flaxseed (linseed), rapeseed (canola), hempseed, walnuts.
Syearidonic acid	Hempseed & animal products
Eicosapentaenoic acid	animal products, in particular fish, some traces in algae.
Docosahexaenoic acid	animal products, in particular fish, some traces in algae.
omega-6 fatty acids	
Linolenic acid	Plant foods, sunflower, safflower, sesame seed, corn, soya beans & walnuts
Gamma-linolenic acid	Borage, evening primrose, hempseed
Arachidonic acid	animal products

High intake of arachidonic acid metabolically diminishes the uptake of the healthier omega-3 fatty acids thus, plant derivative fatty acids are more desirable.

Iron is essential mineral for enzymic reactions in all organisms; consumption is naturally via cereals, soybeans, lentils, Spinach and other plant micronutrients that aid towards optimal health and healthy ageing. Iron is a metabolic catalytic co-enzyme that is stored in the liver, important in hemoglobin for oxygen transportation via the red blood cells. Iron is important in mitochondria for adenosine triphosphate production during aerobic respiration and other metabolic processes.   The iron dependent epigenetic enzyme histone acetyltransferase (see figure 1a & b) facilitates opening of the chromatin gene promoter regions of DNA to enable gene expression. Iron is involved with hemoglobin, phagocytotic white blood cells that assist immunity and diminishes oxidative stress among other functionalities such as the epigenetic regulation of gene expression.

The trace element Selenium modulates the DNA repair system that has anti-inflammatory effect among other epigenetic processes on DNA methylation; Selenium has an preventive effect with respect to chronic diseases such as muscular dystrophy (Hogue et al - 1958) and other undesirable histone modifications due to selenium deficiency; quite often natural food sources do not incorporate adequate selenium due to nutrient-poor-soils, food supplements are advisable via a reasonable multi vitamin and mineral supplement or some other bio-functional foods that incorporates Selenium.

Garlic incorporates DADS (Diallyl Disulfide) that are inhibitors of HDAC (histone deacetylase enzyme, which enables gene expression), 40-60% Diallyl Disulfide is found in garlic of which is metabolize in the liver to inhibitory Allyl Nercaptan (AN) enzyme garlic lowers cholesterol and inhibits platelet aggregation and helps towards optimal health.

Other functional foods that are bioactive nutrient such as Broccoli, cabbage and kale incorporate Sulforaphane which are endogenous antioxidants that help prevent cancer and other health benefits. Green Tea incorporate flavonoid polyphenols, catechin and eipgalloatechin-3-gallate (EGCG) that are biological effectors; The EGCGs (50-70% in green tea) inhibit HATS (histone acetyltransferase enzyme) that inhibit unhealthy gene expression. It has also been shone that EGCG reduce HDAC activity in prostate cancer via the LNCap cells and PC-3 cells, that's suppression of class 1 histone deacetylases carcinogenesis (Thakur, v.s et al - 2005) Green tea has desirable epigenetic effect due to 50-70% EGCGs (see figure 1c & 1d, and appendixes).

Turmeric incorporates curcumin which is a polyphenolic compound that has epigenetic effect; curcumin is an antioxidant that utilizes acetyl-CoA and is a HAT inhibitor. Turmeric is anti-inflammatory due to the HAT inhibiting p300/CBP and HDAC activities (see figure 1b, 1c & 1d) of which, induce anti-inflammatory and anticancer effect (Sharma, et al - 2012). Turmeric also has preventive properties for poor intestinal absorption and preventive properties for type two diabetes via improvement of pancreatic beta-cells functionality. Turmeric is derived from the root rhizomes of the species curcuma longa, that is a member of the ginger classification (see personalized functional foods and Bio-functional-foods).

Table 12 shows functional foods and epigenetic activities that have protective effects against cancer and other diseases

Nutrient	Functional Foods & Source	Epigenetic Activities
Methionine	Sesame seeds, Brazil nuts, fish, peppers, spinach	SAM synthesis
Folic Acid	Leafy vegetables, sunflower seeds, baker's yeast, liver	Methionine synthesis
Vitamin B12	Meat, liver, shellfish, milk	Methionine synthesis
Vitamin B6	Meats, whole grain products, vegetables, nuts	Methionine synthesis
Betaine	Wheat, spinach, shellfish, and sugar beets	Break down the toxic by products of SAM synthesis
Resveratrol	Red wine	Removes acetyl groups from histones, improving health
SAM-e (SAM)	SAM-e (SAM) Popular dietary supplement pill; unstable in food	Enzymes transfer methyl groups from SAM directly to the DNA
Choline	Egg yolks, liver, soy, cooked beef, chicken, veal and turkey	Methyl donor to SAM
Genistein	Soy, soy products	Increased methylation, cancer prevention, unknown mechanism
Sulforaphane	Broccoli	Increased histone acetylation turning on anti-cancer genes

Butyrate	A compound produced in the intestine when dietary fibre is fermented	Increased histone acetylation turning on 'protective' genes, increased lifespan (shown in the lab in flies)
Diallyl sulphide (DADS)	Garlic	Increased histone acetylation turning on anti-cancer genes

Choi, S.W.; Friso, S. Epigenetics: A New Bridge between Nutrition and Health. Adv. Nutr. 2010, 1, 8–16.
Fabiani, R.; Minelli, L.; Bertarelli, G.; Bacci, S. A western dietary pattern increases prostate cancer risk: A systematic review and meta-analysis. Nutrients 2016, 8, 626.

Alcohol effects on epigenetics

Alcohol is a physiological environment factor associated with several diseases due to the cellular toxic effects on many different tissues via acetaldehyde. Acetaldehyde interferes with DNA synthesis and DNA repair system, noted for the underlying effects of lower and upper gastrointestinal tract cancers. Alcohol induces oxidative stress on the liver and other organs, also impairs one-carbon metabolism that regulates availability of methyl groups, resulting in abnormal methyl group transfer thought to the development of various cancers and other associated diseases.

Alcohol has effect on epigenetics via the one-carbon metabolism and DNA methylation that effects gene expressions by modification of the phenotype without alteration of the DNA base sequencing. DNA methylation alters the methyl group of the 5'-carbon of cytosine the occurs at CpG, in dinucleotide sequence in mammalian genome.

DNA methyltransferases (DNMTs) maintains DNMT1 which preserves DNA methylation levels during cellular mitosis. DNMT3A and DNMT3B regulate cytosine methylation sites *(Boland M.J.Christman J.K(2009)*, DNA methylation has a physiological role in normalization of chromosomal imprinting. Thus alcohol interferes with vitamin folate absorption via inhabitation of the one-carbon metabolism directly; folate, a water soluble vitamin B availability is diminish by alcohol intake an intestinal malabsorption thus increased renal excretion due to deficiency of folate or vitamin B9 *(Hamid, A. and Kaur, J(2007)*.

Epigenetic effects of alcohol on the physiology and many associated diseases all occur via mechanisms of DNA methylation and alcohol induced histone modifications on the histone-tail sites, resultant abnormal DNA methylation that has tissue and gene specificity which easily also influenced by diet, age, and genotype in concordance to biomarkers and quantitatively alcohol consumption. Thus, it is reasonable to say alcohol is not advisable (also see appendixes).

Caffeine nutrigenetics

Caffeine is a central nervous system (CNS) stimulant of the methylxanthine class (methylxan-thine alkaloid - 1,3,7-trimethyl xanthine), and isochemically related to the purine adenine and guanine bases of (DNA) and (RNA). Caffeine is contained in seeds, nuts, and leaves of various plants native, most abundant source of caffeine is the seed of Coffee plants, belonging to the botanical family of Rubiaceae, two main species are Coffee arabica and Coffee canephora Caffeine-containing drinks, coffee, tea, and cola, coffee is most frequently used beverage worldwide; caffeine alleviates drowsiness and improves alertness and is the most widely consumed and quite legal mild stimulant.

Caffeine is absorbed through the gastrointestinal tract and metabolized in the liver by cytochrome P450 1A2 (CYP1A2), with resultant metabolites: paraxanthine, theophylline, and bromine. Caffeine levels appear in the bloodstream within 15-45 min, in 1 hour post ingestion of consumption, crossing the blood brain barrier due to its lipid solubility and makes changes in the cerebral fluid via synaptic enzymic activity. Caffeine and metabolites are excreted by the kidneys, and concentrations decrease by 50%-75% within 3-6 hour of consumption.

The main mechanism are adenosine receptor antagonism and secondary effect is inhibition of phosphodiesterase, with accumulation of cyclic AMP and an intensification of the effects of catechol-amines, effects are cognitive response, increased alertness and attention, and in a complex cardiovascular response, increased blood pressure (Tofalo et al., 2016). Many caffeine stimulant effects are mediated by adenosine receptor sub types A1 and A2A, both expressed and differently distributed in human brain, important in sleep-wake regulation (Svenningsson et al., 1997), caffeine acts on the CNS as an adenosine antagonist, though also has effect on substrate metabolism and neuromuscular function (Goldstein et al., 2010).

Figure 1g – shows the interactions of the Circadian Clock, an important part of nutritional regulation.

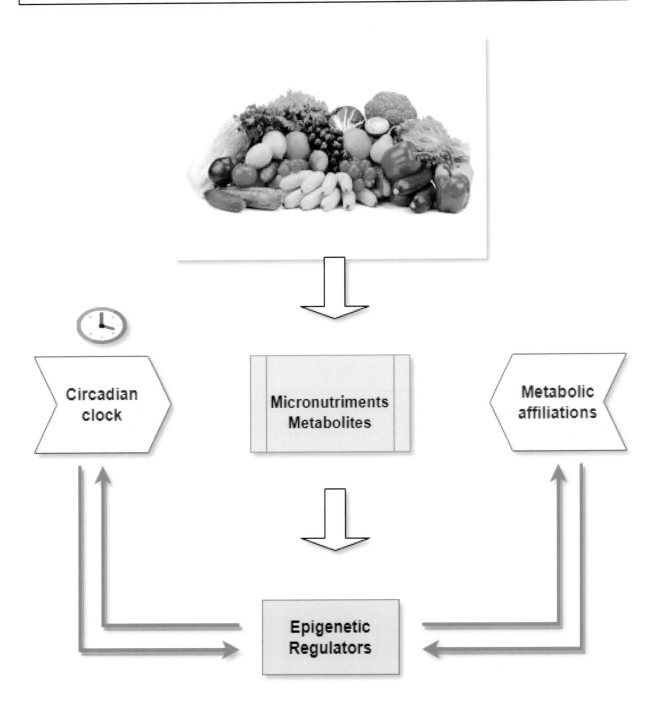

29/04/21

References:

Abbaoui B, Telu KH, Lucas CR, et al. **The impact of cruciferous vegetable isothiocyanates on histone acetylation and histone phosphorylation in bladder cancer.** J Proteomics. 2017;156:94-103.

Boland M.J.Christman J.K. **Mammalian DNA methyltransferases, In Nutrients and Epigenetics.** (eds, Choi, S.W and Frio, S.) Boca Raton, FL: press Taylor & Francis Group, 2009

Chatterjee N, Rana S, Espinosa-Diez C,Anand S. **MicroRNAs in cancer: challenges and opportunities in early detection, disease monitoring and therapeutic agents.** Curr Pathobiol Rep 2017:35-42

Deaton, A.M., Bird, A., 2011. **CpG islands and the regulation of transcription.** Genes Dev 25, 1010e1022.

Duygu B, Poels EM, da Costa Martins PA. **Genetics and epigenetics of arrhythmia and heart failure.** Front Gene 2013:219

Earl R, Thomas PR (eds) (1994) **Opportunities in the nutrition and food sciences: research challenges and the next generation of investigators.** National Academies Press

Fahey JW, Zalcmann AT, Talalay P. **The chemical diversity and distribution of glucosinolates and isothiocyanates among plants.** Phytochemistry. 2001;56(1):551

Fahey JW, Wehage SL, Holtzclaw WD, et al. **Protection of humans by plant glucosinolates: efficiency of conversion of glucosinolates to isothiocyanates by the gastrointestinal microflora.** Cancer Prev Res (Phila). 2012;5(4):603-611.

Fatemi, M., et al., 2005. Foot printing **of mammalian promoters: use of aCpG DNA methyltransferase revealing nucleosome positions at single molecule level.** Nucleic Acids Res 33 (20), e.176

German, E, et el., **Hepatic metabolism of Diallyl Disulfide in rat and man.** Xenobiotica, 2003. 33(12) pp 1185-99]

Gould BS. **Collagen formation and fibogenesis with special reference to the role of ascorbic acid.** International Review of Cytology. 1963:15:301-361.

Goldstein, E.R., Ziegenfuss, T., Kalman, D., et al., 2010. International society of sports nutrition position stand: caffeine and performance. J Int Soc Sports Nutr 7, 5

Hamid, A. and Kaur, J. **Decreased expression of transporters reduces folate uptake across renal absorption surfaces in experimental alcoholism**. J Membbr Biol 220 no. 1-3(2007):69-77

Hecht SS. **Chemoprevention by Isothiocyanates. In:** Kelloff GJ, Hawk ET, Sigman CC, eds. Promising Cancer Chemo preventive Agents, Volume 1: Cancer Chemo preventive Agents Totowa, NJ: Humana Press; 2004:21-35

Hogue, D.E., **vitamin E, selenium and other factors related to muscular dystrophy in limbs.** Cornell nutrition conference for feed manufacturers proceedings, 1958: pp329.

Khattak M. **Biological significance of ascorbic acid (vitamin C) in human health**- A review Pakistan Journal of Nutrition. 2004:3:5-13

Knowles HJ, Ravel RR, Harris AL el al. **Effects of ascorbate on the activity of hypoxa-inducable factor in cancer cells**. Cancer Research. 2003:63:1764-1764. Iacoazzi V, Castegna A, Infantino V, Anddria G. **Mitochondrial DNA methylation as the next generation biomarker and diagnostic tool.** Mool Genet Metabol 2013:110(1-2):25-34

Loche E, Ozanne SE. **Early nutrition, epigenetics and cardiovascular disease.** Curr. Opin Lipidol 2016:449-58

Li, P.et al. p27(Kipl) **stabilisation and G (1) arrest by 1,25-dihydroxyvitamin D(3) in ovarian cancer cells mediated though down-regulation of cyclin E/ cyclindependent kinase 2 and skp1-cullin-F-box protein/skp2 ubiquitin ligase.** J, Biol Chem 279, 2526025267 (2004)

Mazzio EA, Solimin KFA. **Basic concepts of epigenetics impact of environmental signals on gene expression**. Epigenetics 2012:119-30

Piyathilake CJ, Bell WC, Johanning GL et al. **The accumulation of ascorbic acid by squamous cell carcinomas of the lung and larynx is associated globe methylation of DNA**. Cancer. 2000:98:171-176

Svenningsson, P., Nomikos, G.G., Ongini, E., Fredholm, B.B., 1997.Antagonism of adenosine A2A receptors underlies the behaviouralactivating effect of caffeine and is associated with reduced expres-sion of messenger RNA for NGFI-A and NGFI-B in caudate-putamen and nucleus accumbens. **Neuroscience** 79, 753e764.

Sharma, R.A.A.J. Gescher and W.P.Steward, **Curcumin: The story of far.** Eur J Cancer 2005. 41(13): pp1955-68

Traber HG, Stevens JF, **Vitamin C and E: beneficial effects on mechanistic perspective**. Free Radical Biology and Medicine. 2011:51:1000-1013.

Thakur, v.s., k. Gupta, **Green Tea polyphenols cause cell cyclic arrest and apoptosis in prostate cancer by suppressing in class 1 histone deacetylases** carsinogenesis, 2012. 33(2): pp. 377-84.

Thomson C, Bloch AS, Hasler CM, Kubena K, Earl R, Heins J.(1999) **Position of the American dietetic association.** J.Am Diet Assoc 99(10):1278–1285

Tofalo, R., Renda, G., De Caterina, R., Suzzi, G., 2016. Coffee: healtheffects. In: Caballero, B., Finglas, P., Toldra ´, F. (Eds.), **The Encyclopedia of Food and Health**. Academic Press, Oxford,pp. 237e243.

Tonucci LB., Olbrirch Dos Santos KM., Licursi de Oliveerirra L., Rocha Ribeiro SM., Duarte Martino HS. **Clinical applications of probiotics in type 2 diabetes mellitus: a ramderized, double-blind, placebo-controlled study**. Clin Nutr 2017;36(1):85-92

udali S, Guarini P, Morrozzi S, Choi SW, Friso S. **Cardiovascular epigenetics: from DNA methylation to microRNAs.** Mol Aspect. Med 2013:883-901

Van Robertson wb, Schwartz B. Ascorbic **acid and the formation of collagen**, the journal of Biological Chemistry. 953:201:689-696.

Verkerk R, Schreiner M, Krumbein A, et al. **Glucosinolates in Brassica vegetables: the influence of the food supply chain on intake, bioavailability and human health.** Mol Nutr Food Res. 2009;53 Suppl 2: S219.

Weststrate JA, Van Poppel G, Verschuren PM (2002) **Functional foods, trends and future.** Br J. Nutr 88(S2):S233–S235

Wilson CWM, Loh HS. **Vitamin C and colds** The Lancet. 1973:3:5-13.

Wong NW. Chen Y, Chen S, Wang X. **OncomiR: an online reseace for exploring pan-cancer microRNA dysregulation**. Bioinformatics: 2017:713-5

Zhang Y. **Cancer-preventive isothiocyanates: measurement of human exposure and mechanism of action**. Mutat Res. 2004;555(1-2):173-190.

Zang T, Cooper S, Brockdoff N.**The interplay of** *Histone Modifications – writer that read.*
EMBO Rep 2015:16(11):1467-81

Chapter 3

Quantum field biological interactions

The mechanism of functional foods and positive intellectual attitude on epigenetics is via **Quantum field biological interactions** (also see figure 1e - Feynman diagram). Figure 1g - Feynman diagram, (there are an infinite number of Feynman diagrams that are graphical representations of equations).

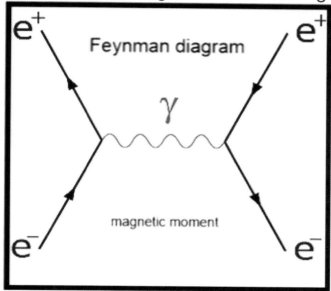

Quantum field biological interactions -The Feynman diagram shows the Electron positron scattering (called the magnetic moment) where two electrons collide to produce a photon Υ, given by two diagrams that represent two integrals that are electrons, and the intermediate photon is virtual Υ is a symbol that carries the quantum numbers of the exchange. The electron scattering exchange is qualitatively even, the two electrons colloid, a photon is emitted and Υ discharges to the other electron fields *(P. Richard - Feynman (1918-1988))*.

Quote: "In biological molecules the electrons *(and all quantum fields)* **are significant, quantum tunnelling and entanglement occur internal to the physiology"** King.J.L(2021)**; though "molecules do not have spherical symmetry"** (Autschach.J., 2021) **although perhaps conform to quantum field theory** (Prof. Tong.D - YouTube) **and super-symmetry.**

Quantum field biological interactions and Pseudocertainty on epigenetics

The **electrodynamic electromagnetic** field interactions, and complexities are quantum field biological interactions and when applicable to physiology are under involuntary subconscious control, the quantum field biological interactions have effect within all organic interactions, and therefore all epigenetic modifications; It would be reasonable to say that all interactions conform to 'natures universal rules' of quantum field electromagnetism as electrons and protons tunnel akin to waves through the DNA and enzymatic molecule structures.

Hypothesis:

The combination of electron spin and quantum field electromagnetism is so highly sensitive, **the act of thought** (pseudocertainty) can modify the quantum field spin of a quark or electron via subconscious electromagnetism (King.JL(2021)) laboratory experimentation will prove this **Hypothesis**; in a similar way to the measurement that modifies the Quarks and electron spin under laboratory conditions, as proven with quantum bitcoin encrypted keys. Quantum bitcoin encryption keys utilize the spin of quantum entangled electron field and the act of measurement via the orientation of the electron spin indicates a 1 or 0; thus, the act of measurement modifies the electron spin to a 1 (up) or 0 (down) status, depending on the initial transmitted electron spin state. Bitcoin quantum entangled encryption keys are considered safer for bank transactions as they <u>do not completely</u> rely on classical programming.

"thought is equal to energy internal to human physiology" (King.J.L(1991)) via **quantum entanglement**, especially with respect to neurology. Neurologically, the sodium and potassium perpetuate the field electromagnetic electrodynamic fields via quantum field biological interactions thus, the electromagnetic chemical transmissions perpetuate (see figure 1e - Feynman diagram) along the nerve fiber (axon) to the synaptic gaps for cerebellum fluid enzymic interactions of which conform to quantum field theory. The above-mentioned quantum field biological interactions are influenced via functional foods, Bio-functional-foods and positive intellectual attitude, effecting epigenetic modifications and therefore immunity which are under involuntary subconscious control. Thus, a conscious positive intellectual attitude has effect of epigenetic enhancement via the subconscious and resultant correct gene expression towards optimum health, though positive or pseudocertainty alone will not achieve optimal healthy ageing in the absence of proper nutrition and exercise.

Telomeres are age related effectors with respect to quantitative cellular replication, and therefore ageing and biological DNA repair system. Each time cell division occurs, the telomeres 'tips' at the end of chromosome diminish as nucleotides erode of the DNA structure and the telomere shortens each cell division, approximately hundred nucleotide telomere repeats must be at the end of chromosome to avoid activation of the biological DNA repair pathways; researchers at Stanford University have developed a new procedure to lengthen chromosomal telomeres, effectively quantitatively increasing cellular division by preventing shortening of the chromosomal 'tips' and extending the biological clock of cellular ageing process; Also Astragalus root have been studied as possible telomerase activators such an extract is TA-65 and vitamin D3 (fish oils) have similar effects of biological clock extension via telomere extension.

The "flow-FISH" test stands for flow cytometry and fluorescence in situ hybridization, that specifically measures the telomere length via blood sample, the flow-FISH test was developed by Canadian researcher Lansdorp, P., (2006) M.D.,Ph.   Stress can diminish telomerase activities thereby shortening the biological clock, the opposite is true for individuals with high telomerase of which adds telomeres thereby extension of biological age via extension of quantitative cellular life, with additional telomeres towards optimal health and healthy ageing (or anti-ageing).

Chapter 4

Future of *epigenetics and synthetic biology*

The future for *epigenetics is further developments in epigenomics and progression of nutrition via enhanced functional foods and Bio-functional foods. Developments toxicology, epidemiology and DoHAD transgenerational among other technological advancement for methods for hydroxy methylation.*

SIRT1 and p53... and the progression of *histone technological advancement i.e., improved DNA sensitivity for TAB sequential LC-MS also 5hmC marks and other, including SIRT1, NAD+ Trans-Resveratrol for anti-ageing or biological age reversal* (Dr D. Sinclair. 2021), also further research with Yamanaker factors (Oct3/4, Sox2, Klf4 ...).

Future advancements of direct detection for *5mC and 5hmC marks is expected, together with detailed understanding of serotonergic marks of serotonlyation. The hormonal functionality of Serotonylation is specific, such as 5-HT in haemostasis and thrombosis is important to possibly prevent and treat haemorrhagic and cardiovascular disorders and beneficial activities with respect to pulmonary hypertension. when large amounts of protein-bound serotonin are found in the blood this suggests the presence of unidentified other serotonylation interactions, suggestive that further research would reveal further proteins, signaling pathways, cellular processes, diseases of serotonylation involvement this is important and necessary research* (Also see Appendix I).

Future advancements in the research specializations of Epigenetic Drift, Germ lineage exposures, single cell epigenetics research will occur as further pioneer technological advancements such as Genome Compilers; Computer simulation of various species, including humans these are controversial advancements in computational epigenetics and synthetic biology have been exponential; the technology has evolved and continues to evolve and evoke bioethics with respect to application of DNA and epigenetic programmable applications.

Bio-Functional-foods

Future of computational *synthetic biology for personalized health will become more refined with possible impacts on the production of* **Bio-Functional-foods that are grown from genetically modified bacteria** resulting in grown functional foods with bioactive enhancements. *Synthetic biology shall have impacts in the long-term future as human genome, perhaps encourage* *population genomic and epigenetic drift though very much in the long-term* future. Epigenetic Clocks for Anti-ageing Treatments, Personalized *synthetic biology will be a significant tool for both gene correction utilising CRISPR system (Cas9 enzyme) and epigenetic modification enhancement providing future Personalized synthetic biology and in the* **long-term** future designer babies utilising Genome Compilers and cloning technologies, although **bioethics** are and will be considerations.

Biomarker methods of measurement

The first transcriptional methods where expression microarrays are of oligonucleotides which are complementary to transcripts whereby fluorescence labelled complementary DNA (cDNA) is generated from RNA and hybridized utilized for transcriptional profiling.

Next generation sequencing data and heterogeneous technology, improving detection of low-level and divers' genetic variations, including single nucleotide variants and complex insertions, deletions, duplications or even inversions. This genomic approach has enabled genetic variants to be studied e.g., genome-wide scans Single nucleotide polymorphisms (SNPs) to identify previous unknown genetic variants that modify nutritional response.

SNP-array based genome typing can offers: WetLab, primary analysis, secondary analysis, tertiary analysis, visualization, nucleic acid extraction and purification library preparations, sequencing, De-multiplexing-based calling, read mapping variant calling, variant annotation variant filtering, and integrative genomics viewer (see Appendix III)

Transcriptomics is utilized to analyze a complete set of RNA transcripts expressed via a cell at specific instance, requires array based high-throughput microarray-based method analysis (or RNA-seq.) identifies the RNA profile using NGS technology. RNA-seq has evolved and is widely used tool in Transcriptomics for RNA or non-coding-RNA profiling. The main advantages of RNA-seq are discovery and quantitative measurements combination is possible, whereas strand-specific protocols are adopted. Sequencing depth or library size results with more quantitative precision though 'transcriptional noise' may occur. SNP-array based Genotyping data have been important for genomic wide association studies and the arrival of affordable NGS technology, one million

SNPs of SNP arrays have been replaced via the entire genomic sequence of three billion nucleotides that challenged bioinformatics with reference to data storage, quality control and analyst. Both nutrigenetic and nutrigenomic studies may require a systems biology approach to interpret the dynamic microbial community. With a increasing the need for validated sets of bioinformatics tools for the acquisition, management, storage, and retrieval of high-throughput datasets, and for important steps of quality control and analysis.

Appendix
Possible chemical pathways of neurogenic metabolism

Patterns of Nutrient/Epigenetic mechanisms of metabolisms

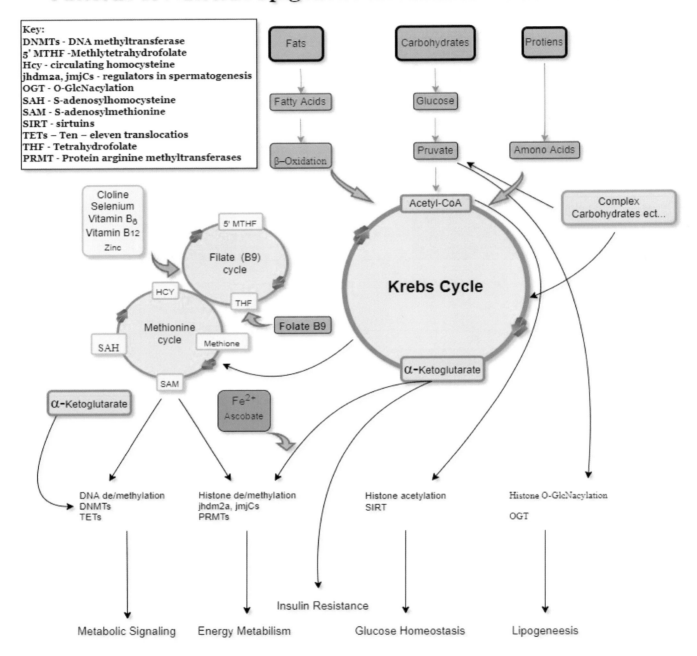

Appendix I

Sirtuins – (SIRT1 - 7) are protein regulatory genes that has anti-ageing properties by switching on longevity genes among other functionalities.

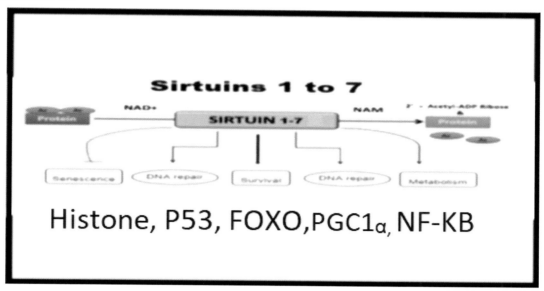

1 - AceCS-1 (acetyl-CoA synthetase) – utilizes Acetyl coenzyme Acetl-coA enzyme of the Krebs-cycle for fatty acid and lipid biosynthesis.	**4 – P53** is a tumor suppressor protein that represses SIRT1 via apoptosis through transcriptional regulation of Autophagy, Senescence, Apoptosis. P53 is also a Biomarker
	5 – PGC-1α is transcription coactivator, mitochondrial biogenesis and also cytoplasmic metabolism, Inflammation and Oxidative Stress.

2 – eNOS – endothelial nitric oxide is a central homeostatic regulator - expression is stimulated via trans-resveratrol that is found in red-grape-skin and Japanese-not-weed – associated with retinal nutrient delivery and functionality in the	The **SIRT1** protein has interactions with NAD+ functionality within nucleic and epithelial cytoplasmic interactions in the heart, liver, skeletal muscles and autophagy (see 1-9).	**6 – FOXOs** - the transcription factor is acetylated in response to stress deacetylation promotes activity in cell cycle inhibition and resistance to oxidative stress. CBP/p300, stimulates its pro-apoptotic activity, both p53dependent or p53-independent.

heart and skeletal muscles.		7 – **CRTC2** - transducers of regulated cAMP (calcium metabolism) response binding protein of transcription
3 - Atgs – Autophagy-related gene or autophagocytosis functionality of lysosome, Yoshinori Ohsum deduced the mechanisms of autophagy during 2016, refers to Cellular degradation.		coactivators, these proteins promote transcriptional cAMP response binding protein of phosphorylated AMP-activated protein kinase sequestered in the liver.
		8 - **SREBP-1** (sterol regulatory element-binding protein 1) is associated with lipogenesis via the insulin stimulated SREBP-1c that enhances glycolysis located in the liver on chromosome 17
		9 – **LXR** - digestive anabolic Liver X Receptors

29/04/21

Appendix II

Quick Reference Guide to *Histone Modifications*

Table 10 - shows the most common histone modifications: -

Histone modification or biomarkers see Appendix III	Functional Location (Ac, Me, P, or Ub) see fugue 1e	Location of histone modification	Marker association
H3K4me1	Activation	Promoters	
H3K4me3	Activation	Gene bodies	
H3K36me3	Activation	Gene bodies	
H3K79me2	Activation	enhancers, promoters	
H3K9Ac	Activation	enhancers, promoters	
H3K4me2	Activation	enhancers, promoters	Embryonic development epigenetic memory
H3K27Ac	Activation	enhancers, promoters	
H4K16Ac	Activation	Biological Repetitive sequences	
H3K27me3	Repression	Promoters, gene rich regions	Embryonic development epigenetic memory
H3K9me3	Repression	Biological repeats, telomeres, per centromeres	
Gamma H2A.X	DNA replication DNA double strand breaks		
H3S10P	DNA replication	Mitotic chromosomes	

Appendix III

Computational gene mapping and *biomarkers*

Appendix III shows an example of computational gene mapping showing gene *biomarkers or SNPs, researchers have found SNPs may help predict an individual's response to certain drugs, susceptibility to environmental factors such as toxins,*

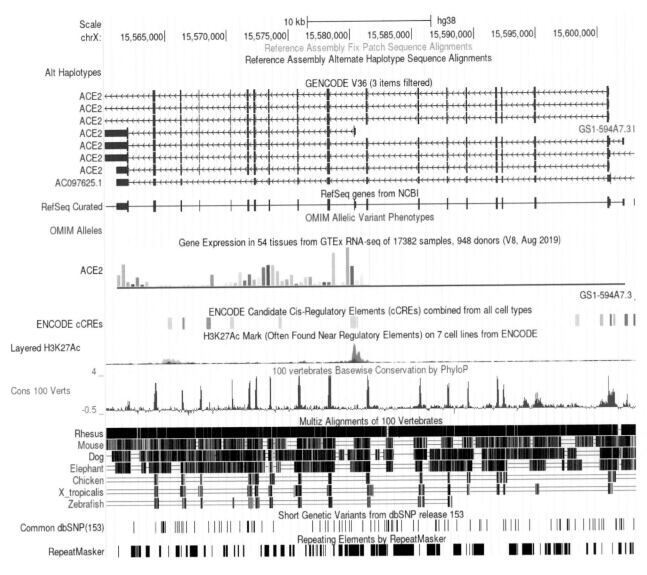

and risk of developing particular diseases. SNPs can also be used to track the inheritance of disease genes within families. SNPs may help predict an individual's response to certain drug types and susceptibility to environmental factors such as toxins, and the risk of developing particular

diseases. *SNPs can also be used to track the* **inheritance of disease gene** *biomarkers within families though epigenetics is dynamic thus inheritance is not always applicable due to systems of biological age reversal.*

Bio-Functional-foods are grown from genetically modified bacteria, fungi and algae - utilising synthetic biology

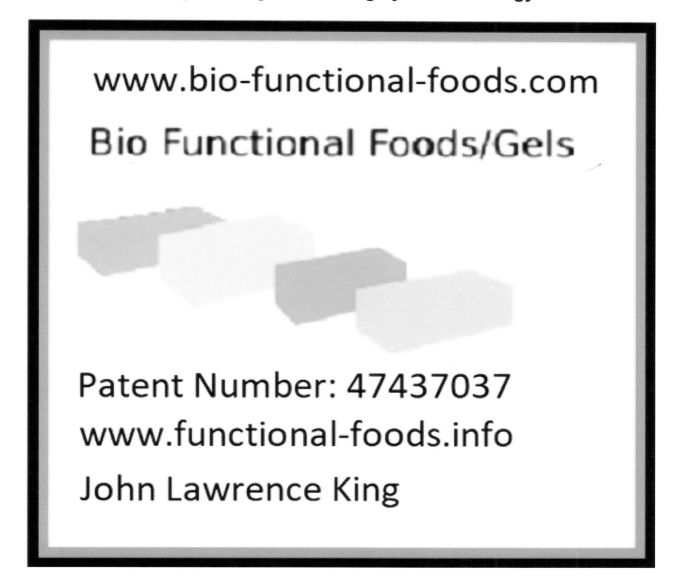

Re: to feed populations after/during droughts or floods and supermarket supplies

This was posted to the Botswana government and Whitehouse and Chinese government re: to feed global populations after or during droughts or floods.

Functional foods are foods grown from bacteria, fungi and algae (utilising synthetic biology); grown under laboratory conditions on an industrial scale. The functional foods should contain, NAD+, Sirtuins, trans-resveratrol, protein, minerals, vitamins and other health beneficial ingredients. The tofu-like-jelly-blocks of functional foods would be in different colours to represent different nutrients that have both nutritional and health benefits, perhaps complement or replacement of fruit and vegetables due to long shelf-life (1 year); also, to feed populations after/during droughts or floods and dessert environments.

I have written a book: nutrition, functional foods and epigenetics and shall publish in the future.

John Lawrence king

Appendix IV
Epigenetic resources

There are more than 100 papers per year on histone methylation and acetylation and plenty of internet resources: -

IHEC – international Human *epigenome Consortium* - **HEC Data Portal IHE makes available comprehensive sets of reference epigenomics relevant to health and disease via data portal-** *http://ihec-epigenome s.org/* the objectives of the Assay Standards Working Group is twofold: to define the assays required for three distinct classes of reference *epigenome, and to define standardized protocols and quality control metrics for each assay.*

UCSC - *epigenome project -* *https://www.genome.ucsc.edu* On June 22, 2000, UCSC and the other members of the International Human Genome Project consortium completed the first working draft of the human genome assembly, forever ensuring free public access.

The following tools and utilities created by outside groups may be helpful:(a)

BEDOPS - A highly scalable and easily parallelizable genome analysis tools - A

selection of tools for a wide-range of genomics analysis tasks

(b)   bwtool - A command-line utility for bigWig files

(c)   CrossMap - A program for genome coordinate conversion between different assemblies

(d)   CruzDb - Python package to load genome annotations from our servers

(e)   libBigWig - A C library to read bigWig files, without a dependency on our source code

(f)   MakeHub - Python tool to build assembly hub files for new genomes

(g)   RTracklayer - R package to import genome annotations from our databases

(h)   trackhub - Python package to manage files in our trackDb format

(i)   twobitreader - Python package to open 2bit genome sequence files

(j)   ucsc-genomes-download - Python package to download genome sequences from our servers

(k)   WiggleTools - C++ Unix command-line tool to work with bigWig files: combine, merge, scale, aggregate and many other operations

Deep blue - *epigenetic data server - deepblue.mpi-inf.mpg.de/*   ***The DeepBlue** Epigenomic Data Server provides a central data access hub for large collections of epigenomic data. It organizes the data from different sources using controlled vocabularies and ontologies. The data is stored in our server, where the users can access the data programmatically or by our web interface*

Epigenie – informally informative – ***https://epigenie.com****,* *Epigenetic regulatory cascades can be complex affairs…a recent chromatin effector self-regulatory organisation.*

Toolbox Genomics kits – test t*hat shows epigenetic health-toolbox Genomics - DNA Test Kits & Panels For Licensed ...www.32andMe.com...* **https://www.toolboxgenomics.com** *a variety of DNA tests for clients, with different options for both licensed healthcare practitioners as well as other health & wellness professionals.*

Science Journals available on *epigenetics: -*

➤   epigeneticsepigenomics
➤   environmental *epigenetics*
➤   clinical *epigeneticsepigenetics insightsepigenetics and chromatinepigenetics and epigenomics...*
➤   this list would be infinite with YouTube as approaching 2021+

29/04/21

References and further internet research:

→ sheeky   science   -   SIRT1   go   down   in   ageing   &   senescence?   -   Bing   video
   https://www.bing.com/videos/search
→ p53 - Bing images https://www.bing.com
→ PGC-1α, Inflammation, and Oxidative Stress: An Integrative View in Metabolism
→ https://www.hindawi.com/journals/omcl/2020/1452696/
→ Enforced PGC-1α expression promotes CD8 T cell fitness, memory formation and antitumor
   immunity lxr- anabolism - Bing images https://www.bing.com/images/search?
→ Cellular & Molecular Immunology (www.nature.com)
→ www.researchgate.net
→ www.abcam.com
→ Functional Nutrition Alliance

Glossary

- **5-hmC - 5-Hydroxymethyl<u>cytosine</u>** *(see Ten-eleven transferase (TET) enzymes)*

- **5-mC - 5-Methyl<u>cytosine</u>** *(see Ten-eleven transferase (TET) enzymes)*

- **5' MTHF -Methlytetrahydrofolate** *– active folic acid, involved in serotonin and methionine production and also DNA synthesis.*

- **Acetylation** *- influence transcriptional regulation and expression with lysine residues, describes a reaction that inserts an acetyl functional group into a biological compound. The opposite biological reaction is called* **deacetylation** *that removes the acetyl group. Acetylation can alter gene expression epigenetically.*

- **Autophagy** *– replenishment of cells (degradation) for heather cells.*

- **Crotonylation** *is a reversible modification via crotonyl transferases (***writers***) and decrotonylases (***erasers***). Crotonylation has overlapped acyl-transferases and de-acylases with acetylation and other types of histone acylations at site 25, 30 and also overlapped modification sites on histones at 29, 31. additional epigenetic modification on histones, crotonylation also occurs in histone proteins 25, 26, 27, 28 and participates metabolic pathways such as acetylation 29 on the histone complex. These findings suggest that crotonylation is a global PTM with a complex interplay with other acylations Lysine crotonylation on histones is a recently identified post-translational modification and been demonstrated to associate with active promoters to directly stimulate transcription.*

- **Citrullination** *- citrullination is a novel arginine-directed post-translational modification resultant in permanent change in the referenced protein. Peptidyl arginine deiminases mediate calcium-dependent deamination of the guanidino group of* **arginine side chains.** *Citrullination is a facilitator modifying known "self-antigens" to foreign, unrecognized proteins, vulnerable immunity. Citrullination is a* **general regulatory mechanism that occurs during apoptosis;** *Citrullination is also* **part of normal physiology**, *for example, citrullination of trichohyalin in the* **hair follicle**, *myelin* basic protein, **histones in the nucleus**, and **keratin in the nails and skin**.

- **Chromosomes** are comprised of chromatins (see histones, octamers, nucleosome and DNA)
- **CRISPR/Cas9** is a system for gene editing, utilising Cas9 bacterial enzyme that utilizes a guide RNA molecule to find and modify specific nucleotide sequences in the eukaryotic genome.

- **DADS** - Diallyl Disulfide and Allyl Nercaptan (AN) are both **inhibitors** of HDAC activity (see HDAC)

- **Demethylation** is a pathway resultant in the removal of a methyl molecular group (CH_3), most **demethylation** results in the replacement of a methyl group by a hydrogen atom, with a loss of one carbon and two hydrogen atoms, the counterpart of **demethylation** is methylation.

- **DNMTs - DNA methyltransferase** – family of enzymes that regulate epigenetic affiliates.

- **Genome Compiler** or DNA compiler – is an all-in-one platform for genetic engineering and synthetic biology provides a set of comprehensive tools for DNA design and visualization, and a seamless DNA ordering via all-in-one software. The Materials Box inside DNA compiler consists of sequences from Addgene, Sigma Aldrich, Synberc, Lucigen, iGEM, Plasmapper; it is possible to query the NCBI database from within and instantly import your data into the Materials Box directly from DNA Compiler and post the compiled product to an organization for production of the complied genomic, bacteria or fungi basted product.

- **DNA is a negatively charged helical structure** due to the phosphate groups in its phosphate-sugar backbone, an octamer histone complex coil up tightly to form nucleosome, as the sum of nucleosol histone complexes is positively charged proteins that adhere to negatively-charged DNA and form complexes called nucleosomes.

- **DNA methylation** *(CpG and non-CpG) – gene sequencing that is enriched at CpG (a methyl group (CH_3–) is introduced); an additional methyl groups is component of bases of DNA (see methylation)*

- **Electron** *- An electron is a negatively charged (though sometime positive called a cation subatomic particle. Electrons can be either free or bound to the nucleus of an atom. Electrons spherical shells the represent energy levels; the charge on a single electron is considered as the unit electrical charge.*

- **Epigenome** *epigenomics is the analysis of genome-wide consequences of epigenetic modifications across many genes in cells or entire organism. The Human Epigenome/Genome Project is an international collaboration 'to identify, catalogue and interpret genome-wide epigenetic methylation patterns of all human genes.*

- **Epigenetic Drift** *- the genomic sequence does not change over time, however, epigenetic marks, and methylation are variable histone modifications underlying gene expression and control differentiates cell types, the epigenetic patterns are established early in development. There is a highly developed mathematical theory of how quasi-neutral mutations may behave in populations.*

- **Epigenetic regulation** *– of transcription comprises of three - Histone modifications, DNA methylation, and non-coding RNA.*

- **Epigenetics project road map** *– shows chromatin computational maps in the UCSC genome project browser - indicates RNA transcription gene cluster(mark) showing states and events of different tissue types.*

- **Epigenetics** *- The study of heritable meiotic and/or miotic changes in gene expression and/or repression functionalities that are not resultant of changes in DNA sequence; subtle chemical changes such as methylation of the nucleotide cytosine in gene promoter sequences or acetylation of the histone proteins with which DNA is structurally associated.; or: heritable stabilized phenotype of structural chromosomal modifications effecting histone octamer complex methylation and acetylation involved in tissue specific patterns t- hat register and signal heritable gene expression* *without sequential DNA modifications. gH2AX assay Phosphorylated gH2AX is a protein that accumulates at epigenetic sites that is detected by fluorescent antibodies, used to determine the amount of chromosomal strand breaks within a nucleus.*

- **Gene locus** *is the specific physical location of a gene or DNA sequence on a chromosome, the plural of locus is -* **loci**

- **Genome** *– total genetic material within a biological cell or system.*

- **GlcNAcylation** *- O-GlcNAcylation is the attachment of O-linked N-acetyl glucosamine (O-GlcNAc) moieties to cytoplasmic nuclear mitochondrial proteins is a regulatory post-translational modification, that involves cytoplasmic cellular processes with nuclear proteins and addition of OGlcNAc to proteins that are catalyzed by O-GlcNAc transferase, and its removal is catalyzed by O-GlcNAc–selective N-acetyl-β-dglucosaminidase.*

- **HAT** *- Histone acetyltransferases catalyze the transfer of an acetyl group from acetyl coenzyme A, while histone deacetylases (HDAC) perform the antagonistic state of removing the acetyl group. Histone acetylation has an important role in the modulation of chromatin condensation and transcriptional regulation.*

- **HDAC** *are enzymes which remove acetyl groups from lysine residues in the tail region of histone/octamer complexes or nucleosomes. Through this mechanism, HDAC are involved in the modification of chromatin architecture and govern the repression of oncogenes, tumor suppressors, and inflammatory genes (de Ruijter et al., 2003), garlic contains 40-60% DADS (Diallyl Disulfide).*

- **Histones** *- are family of small positively charged proteins (amino acid residues such as lysine and arginine) are termed H1, H2A, H2B, H3, and H4 (Van Holde, 1988) that form an octameter, with linker proteins making a nucleosome involved in regulation...*

- **Histone-tail modifications** *- Histone-tail modifications are transactional epigenetics that undergo events via - acetylation, phosphorylation, or methylation, these three are necessary to allow the activity of the* chromatin remodeling complex. Methylation activates or represses gene expression depending on which residue is methylated; Methylation of histone methyltransferases (HMTs), of Lysine SET domain containing (histone tails) and Non-SET domain containing (histone core octamer)

- **Histone acetylation** – occurs on the ε-amino lysine residue and promotes DNA unfolding – CoA (acetyl coenzyme A) and lysine where HAT (histone acetyltransferase enzyme, inhibits gene expression - i.e. repression for immunological defense) and HDAC (histone deacetylase enzyme, HDAC enables nucleic gene expression), n-butyrate is a HDAC inhibitor where HATs are co-activators during transcription. HATs categories are: GCN5, MYST(MOZ), P300/CBP and SRC/p160 of the nuclear receptor co-activator family. Histone and non-histone proteins are catalyzed via HATs. Reversible histone acetylation catalyzed via HATs and HDATs also histone acetylation can inhibit H1-mediated salt insolubility assisting salt solubility concentrations that effects binding and relaxation of DNA coils on the nucleosomal structure. Thus, HATS and HDAC are involved in control gene expression switching gene expression off or on. This effect is consistent with the expected large reduction in electron density on the amino nitrogen upon acetylation thus, making coordination with the coenzyme copper much less strong; the structure of histones shows the patterns of histone acetylation and DNA methylation are quite precise and important mechanisms for epigenetic alteration of gene expression. (See acetylation, HATs, HDAC, histone methylation and figure 1a, 1b and figure 1d).

- Hcy - circulating homocysteine – high levels in the blood are undesirable due to coagulation.

- **Histone methylation** cause local formation of chromatin, which is reversible also can activate or suppress gene expression in accordance to different lysine dependent states (i.e. Mono-methyl, Di-methyl, or Trimethyl (binds the DNA coils around the octamers); The demethylated function is in reverse releasing the DNA coils during transcription. There are **seven** transcriptional regulatory core histone modifications on the 3 histone-tail that is:– 2 active promoters (**H3K9ac**, **H3K4me3**), 2 enhancer promoters (**H3K4me1** (stem cell line), **H3K27ac**), 1 transcribed gene bodies (**H3K36me3**), 1 polycomb promoters(**H3K27me3**), 1 heterochromatin (**H3K9me3**) it is possible to define chromatin profile states(marks) of the genome via the seven histone-tail modification marker state (see acetylation, histone acetylation, HATs, HDAC, and figure 1a, 1b and figure 1d) **Histone modifications** – mark transcriptional events that are ether – active, repressed, or poised states (see figure 1d).

- **Isomerization -** Isomerism definition is compounds which have same molecular formula but differ in reverse arrangement of atoms known as isomers classification of isomerism. There are two main types of isomerism: - structural isomerism and stereoisomerism.

- **Immunity -** The ability of an organism to resist a particular infection or toxin by the action of specific antibodies or hypersensitive white blood cells.

- **Lysine methylation** – enable transcriptional regulatory binding sites for core histone modificatory co-activators on histone tails (see histone methylation).

- **Methylation -** A chemical reaction in which a methyl group (CH_3-) is introduced in a molecule. A particular example is the replacement of a hydrogen atom by a methyl group DNA methylation is a common molecular alteration in colorectal cancer cells.

- **Microbiota** – (microfauna and microflora) The smallest organisms, comprising Bacteria, Fungi, and algae. Microbiota are found in the lungs, stomach, intestinal tract and colon.

- **Neutron** consist of 1 up quark and 2 down quarks. Also, an elementary particle that has no charge, with a mass slightly greater than that of a proton, and spin of a ½, a component of the nuclei of all atoms except those of hydrogen (see quark & protons).

- **Nucleosome core complex is made from an octamer** that is a eight histone protein complex, at the center of a nucleosome consists of two copies of the four core histone proteins (H2A, H2B, H3 and H4), involved in chromatin folding and co-factor recruitment (see figure 1a, 1b, 1d).

- **OGT - O-GlcNacylation** – *enzymic post-translational regulator with TET2 interactions to produce hydroxy methyl cytosine regulating transcription.*

- **Phenotype** *is the total physical gene expression, different genotypes may result from different Phenotype, mutations can cause changes in phenotype.*

- **Positive intellectual attitude** – *an approach that can be advantageous towards optimal health, i.e., healthy-lifestyle-choices towards exercise and intake of healthy nutrition (also see figure 1c - Feynman diagram and Quantum field biological interactions and functional foods on epigenetics).*

- **Phosphorylation - is a** *biochemical process that involves addition of phosphate to an organic compound. Examples are the addition of phosphate to glucose producing glucose monophosphate with addition of phosphate to adenosine diphosphate (ADP) to form adenosine triphosphate (ATP). Phosphorylation is carried out utilising the enzyme phosphotransferases or kinases.* **Phosphorylated gH2AX** *is a protein that accumulates at sites of DNA breaks, detection via fluorescent antibodies that is used to determine the quantity of DNA strand breaks within a nucleus* **Phosphorylation regulates** *ubiquitylation.*

- **PRMT - Protein arginine methyltransferases** – *mediate protein(s) substrate methylation of arginine residues, involved in T-lymphocyte activation and gluconeogenesis.*

- **Proton** - *a proton is a subatomic stable particle with mass defined as positive charge made from three quarks (2 up & 1 down). The atomic number is the number of protons within an atom, the nucleus of every atom contains protons, both protons and neutrons are found in the atom (see quark & neutron).*

- **Ubiquitylation** – *(or ubiquitination) is an enzymatic process involves the bonding of a ubiquitin protein to a substrate protein, Ubiquitin contains conserved sequence of 76 amino acids and linked via covalently bonded proteins proteasomes that promotes apoptosis of the cell; the ubiquitous protein proteasomes is present in all eukaryotic cells. Ubiquitylation* regulated post-translational modification of proteins of ubiquitin molecule, attached to a lysine amino acid in the **Degradation** of p53 promoted by E3 ubiquitin ligase ITCH via ubiquitylation at the **N-terminal border of SAM** (methyl group donor) **domain** of the p53 [alpha] isoforms; the process of **ubiquitination** can be **reversed** through the action of **deubiquitinase** enzymes, by altering the bond between ubiquitin molecule and substrate protein (see phosphorylation**)**.

- **repression** – inhibits epigenome gene expression, the epigenome defense mechanism (ability to switch genes off and on) that co-evolved within invertebrates.

- **SAM -** S-Adenosyl-methionine is a methyl group donor, a substrate that product is SAH.

- **SAH - S-adenosylhomocysteine** – a protein that has a product of SAH into homocysteine and adenosine.

- **SIRT1 – Sirtuins - see Appendix I**

- **Serotonylation** is a receptor independent signaling mechanism, a process for exocytosis of thrombocytes of the blood platelets via serotonlyation of small GTPases such as Rab4 and RhoA. Serotonylation activates of serotonin 5-hydroxytryptamine (that is a neurotransmitter) during intracellular processes that have lasting effects of covalent bonds within enzymes. The enzymes attach to the serotonin on glutamine residues, this signaling mechanism utilizes transglutaminase antibody enzyme for the creation of glutamylamide bonds. Serotonylation is through small GTPases the process by which serotonin controls release of pancreatic insulin from beta cells for the regulation of blood glucose levels. Thus, defects in transglutaminase lead to glucose intolerance, small GTPases are involved, and also regulate vascular aorta smooth muscles. serotonylation modifying proteins are also integral to cytoskeleton via alpha-actin, beta-actin, gamma-actin and myosin heavy chains. Serotonin is also a regulator of mood, appetite, and sleep cognitive functions, memory and learning.

- **Small GTPases** - *are tightly regulated molecular switches that make binary on/off through controlled usage of GTP activation and hydrolysis of GTP to GDP that is inactivation.*

- **Subconscious** *is part of the mind that controls involuntary movement and automatic-immunity.....whilst a higher percentage the brain is functioning on alpha waves; the conscious is part of the mind that controls voluntary movement and conscious thoughts, whilst mostly higher percentage functioning on beta waves, though there are other measurable wave frequencies.*

- **Supersymmetry** *is an extension of the Standard Model that predicts a partner particle (referred to as anti-matter) for each particle in the Standard Model (see Standard Model)*

- **Standard Model** – *a mathematical description of the elementary particles (of fields) of matter and electromagnetic, weak, and strong forces by which they interact (see Supersymmetry).*

- **Sumoylation**, *is a post-translational modification that attaches the SUMO protein to intended proteins regulating activity, function, subcellular localization and stability (Sumoylation Inhibits TAK-981)*

- **Synthetic biology** – *A scientific field that draws on principles of engineering to create new biological parts, devices, or systems to redesign or improve natural biological systems; The capability to make DNA polymers with specific base sequences that behave as genes. These DNA polymers consist of various small DNA sequences that are programmed together (via amino acid, DNA or protein computational program compilers) by homologous recombination to produce functional genes with required genomic and epigenetic health benefit properties to achieve healthy ageing or age reversal (Synthetic biology is also used with mice, yeast, bacteria and fungi).*

- **Ten-eleven transferase (TET) enzymes** – *TET1 or TET2 is found in the embryonic stem cells, while TET3 is found in the stem cells; the TETs are expressed* **ubiquitously** *in differentiated cells, (TET1) is a DNA demethylation enzyme associated with tumorigenesis and biological* *process via catalysis and hydroxylation of DNA (5-methylcytosine (5mC) to 5-hydroxymethylcytosine (5hmC), further catalyze oxidation of 5hmC to 5-formylcytosine (5fC) and then to 5-carboxycytosine (5caC). There are interactions between TET, active DNA demethylation (of DNA base cytosine), transcription, genomic instability, and the DNA damage/repair response.*

- **Telomeres** *are protective tips at the ends of chromosomes, during cellular division, the tips shorten and over time, the telomeres become too short to sustain cell division and the cell become senescent. Other influences include age, stress, poor lifestyle choices and exposure to environmental toxins, it is essential to maintain telomere length.* **Telomerase** *is naturally occurring enzyme that lengthens telomeres and prevents shortening thereby* **extending the biological clock with telomere extension therapeutic techniques.**

- **THF – Tetrahydrofolate** *– one-carbon group carrier involved in amino and nucleic acid biosynthesis and thymidine precursor in synthetic pathways*

- **Quark** *- any of a number of subatomic particles carrying a fractional electric charge, it takes three quarks (1 up 2 down held together by gluons) to make a proton (see proton & neutron).*

Bibliography

Adapted graphics: Google and wallpaperflare

Autschach.J., **(2021); Quantum Theory for Chemical Applications. Oxford University Press.** ISBN-9780190920807

Amstrong.L, (2014) **Epigenetics** Garland Science. ISBN-978-0-8153-6511-2

Bentley N., Dr, **(1996); lecture notes from NESCOT** (Biochemist)
Burton, R., Dr, **(1996); lecture notes from NESCOT** (Geneticist)
Collins, P., Dr, **(1996); lecture notes from NESCOT** (Biochemist)
Hodgson., J, Dr, **(1996); lecture notes from NESCOT** (Cell Biologist)
Kurowski., M., Dr, **(1996); lecture notes from NESCOT** (Cambridge, Microbiologist)
Nichols, R., Dr, **(1996); lecture notes from NESCOT** (Virologist)
Shinabaun., R, Dr, **(1996); lecture notes from NESCOT** (Physiologist)
Ware., D, Dr, **(1996); lecture notes from NESCOT** (OU, Mycologist)

Cévoli and Carlota Castro Espín and Virginie Béraud and Genevieve Buckland and RaulZamora Ros, - **An Overview of Global Flavonoid Intake and its Food Sources**, Flavonoids, (2017), (17),(10.5772/67655) doi.org/10.5772/67655

Choi, S.W.; Friso, S. Epigenetics: **A New Bridge between Nutrition and Health.** Adv. Nutr. 2010, 1, 8–16.

Darnel, J., Baltimore. D., Matsudaira.D., ZipurskyL.S.,Anald.B., Logish.H.,**(2000); Molecular Cell Biology.** Pub. W.H. Freemen and company. ISBN-0-7167-3136-3

Fabiani, R.; Minelli, L.; Bertarelli, G.; Bacci, S. **A western dietary pattern increases prostate cancer risk**: A systematic review and meta-analysis. Nutrients 2016, 8, 626.

Ferguson B.S., (2019) **Nutritional Epigenetics *Academic*** Press. ISBN- 978-0-12-816843-1.

Fung, T.; Hu, F.B.; Fuchs, C.; Giovannucci, E.; Hunter, D.J.; Stampfer, M.J.; Colditz, G.A.; Willett, W.C. **Major dietary patterns and the risk of colorectal cancer in women.** Arch. Intern. Med. 2003, 163, 309–314.

Garland Science (2008) **The Cell.** 5th ed.

Güçlü Üstündağ, Özlem & Mazza, Giuseppe. (2007). **Saponins: Properties, Applications and Processing.** Critical reviews in food science and nutrition. 47. 231-58. 10.1080/10408390600698197.

Hanson, J., Dr, **(1998); lecture notes from University of Bolton** (*Biologist*)

Stannard, S **(2003); lecture notes from University of Bolton** *(ITT-Tutor)*
Ho. E., Domann.F.,**(2020) Nutrition and Epigenetics**. Press. Taler & Francis, FL. ISBN-13: 978-0-367-65899-1

King.J.L., **(2021); Nutrition, Functional-foods and epigenetics an introduction., pp 1,2,7,10. first edition, Publisher Lulu & Amazon. ISBN: - 10 : 1915463521; ISBN-13 :** 978-1915463524 **Email address: johnlawrenceking1@gmail.com**

Kurowsk, M., Dr, **(1996); lecture notes from NESCOT (**Cambridge Dr of Microbiology)

Marechal.Y.,**(2007); The Hydrogen Bond and the Water Molecule**. The physics and chemistry of water, aqueous and bio media. ISBN-10-444-55930-2

Merched, Aksam & Corcuff, Jean-Benoît. (2016). **Nutrigenomics and Nutrigenetics: The Basis of Molecular Nutrition.** 10.1016/B978-0-12-801816-3.00003-0.

Miller., Spoolman (1998). **Living in the Environment: Principles, Connections and Solutions** (Wadsworth Biology Series) 1SBN: 0-534-23898-X

Mohanty, Sujata & Singhal, Kopal. (2018). **Functional Foods As Personalised Nutrition: Definitions and Genomic Insights**. 10.1007/978-981-13-1123-9_22.

Mozafari M.R.,Mohebbi M., Fathi M..(2012) **Nanoencapsulation of food ingredients using lipid based delivery systems** *Trends in Food Science and Technology*, 23 (1) ,pp.13-27.

Nasr, Nasr. (2015). **Applications of Nanotechnology in Food Microbiology.** International Journal of Current Microbiology and Applied Sciences. 4. 846-853.

Olmedilla-Alonso (OR Olmedilla), Begoña. (2017). **Carotenoids: content in foods, in diet and bioavailability**.. 10.13140/RG.2.2.20315.98080.

Panche, Archana & Diwan, Arvind & Chandra, S. (2016). **Flavonoids: An overview.** Journal of Nutritional Science. 5. 10.1017/jns.2016.41.

Raffaele De, C., Alfredo J, Kohlmeier MM. (2020) **Principles of Nutrigenetics and Nutrigenomics Fundamentals of Individualized Nutrition:** ISBN:978-0-12-804572-5

Richard.,P.,(2011);**- Feyman, Six Not-So-Easy Pieces.** ISBN: 078-0-465-02528-2 *(also introduced the Feyman diagrams in 1948)*

Sekhon BS. (2014) **Nanotechnology in agri-food production: an overview. Nanotechnology, Science and Applications.** ;7:31-53. DOI: 10.2147/nsa.s39406.

Sinclair. D. Pro.Dr (2021). - **Lifespan** and You Tube - Biological Age Reversal (**Transresveratrol**) Researcher *et el.*

Tong.D. Profs **(2020) - YouTube - Quantum field theory**

Wai-Yee Fung, Kay-Hay Yuen, and Min-Tze Liong (2011) **Agrowaste-Based Nanofibers as a Probiotic Encapsulant: Fabrication and Characterization** Journal of Agricultural and Food Chemistry 59(15), 8140-8147 DOI: 10.1021/jf2009342

Walsh S. (2003) **Plant Based Nutrition and Health**. ISBN:0-907337-26-0

Vuong, Quan & Stathopoulos, Costas & Nguyen, Minh & Golding, John & Roach, Paul. (2011). **Isolation of Green Tea Catechins and Their Utilization in the Food Industry.** Food Reviews International. 27. 227-247. 10.1080/87559129.2011.563397.

Index